Revolutionizing
Women's Healthcare

Revolutionizing Women's Healthcare

The Feminist Self-Help Movement in America

HANNAH DUDLEY-SHOTWELL

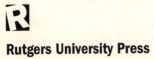

Rutgers University Press

New Brunswick, Camden, and Newark, New Jersey, and London

Library of Congress Cataloging-in-Publication Data

Names: Dudley-Shotwell, Hannah, author.
Title: Revolutionizing women's healthcare : the feminist self-help movement in America /
Hannah Dudley-Shotwell.
Description: New Brunswick : Rutgers University Press, [2020]
Identifiers: LCCN 2019018818 | ISBN 9780813593029 (paperback) |
ISBN 9780813593036 (cloth)
Subjects: LCSH: Women's health services—United States. | Women's health services—
Political aspects—United States. | Feminism—Health aspects—United States.
Classification: LCC RA564.85 .D85 2020 | DDC 362.1082—dc23
LC record available at https://lccn.loc.gov/2019018818

A British Cataloging-in-Publication record for this book is available from the British Library.

www.rutgersuniversitypress.org

Manufactured in the United States of America

For Caroline Marigold

Contents

Abbreviations

BPI	Be Present, Inc.
BWHI	Black Women's Health Imperative
CR	consciousness raising
EGC	Emma Goldman Clinic
FWHC	Feminist Women's Health Center
NACB	Native American Community Board
NAWHERC	Native American Women's Health Education Resource Center
(N)BWHP	(National) Black Women's Health Project
NOW	National Organization for Women
NWHN	National Women's Health Network
OBOS	*Our Bodies, Ourselves*
OM	Ovulation Method
PTP	Pelvic Teaching Program
WATCH	Women Acting Together to Combat Harassment
WCHC	Women's Community Health Center
WCSC	Women's Community Service Center
ZANU	Zimbabwe African National Union

**Revolutionizing
Women's Healthcare**

Introduction

A widely shared feminist circular from 1971 offered this representation of a woman's typical visit to her doctor:

> I've got an itch. So I gotta call the doctor. When I call, the receptionist asks, "What's wrong?" and proceeds to make an appointment from one to two weeks hence. So I wait. . . . Often the bladder becomes infected while waiting for the appointment interval to pass. Finally, I get to see this physician, and [he] comments on examining me, draped in a sheet so that I couldn't watch even if I wanted to, "Usual female infection. Take the antibiotic prescription and come back in two weeks." $$$ When I ask him if I can see what the infection looks like, the physician is appalled at the idea. "You shouldn't worry your little head about this kind of thing. After all, isn't that what I'm here for?["] So I return in 2 weeks $$$$, and maybe it's cleared and maybe it isn't. Another kind of antibiotic is prescribed and another appointment is made $$$. I again ask for specific information about the infection, and by now the answer usually comes back in Greek (which I am obviously not very fluent in).[1]

The self-help movement emerged in the 1960s as a response to medical encounters like this one. This movement became a critical part of feminist activism in the late 1960s as a range of women's health activists criticized and drew attention to the ways that the authority to make decisions about a woman's health and reproduction typically lay with male physicians. Most activists had personal experiences resembling the one above; some had seen worse, including the horrors of botched abortions and nonconsensual sterilization. These activists taught themselves skills usually performed by doctors, a practice they began to call "self-help" in the early 1970s. These early efforts generated an entire movement of women who appropriated their own bodies and minds as tools of knowledge. Women who promoted these efforts held disparate and sometimes competing philosophies about *how* to practice self-help, but all agreed that taking power over their bodies and minds away from physicians and holding it in their own hands was a crucial element of feminism. Tired of feeling as if they had no control over their own bodies, for these women, feminism was literally about health versus sickness. For many, it was utterly transformative.

In the 1960s and 1970s, America experienced unprecedented social turmoil. Leftist activists took to the streets, the media, the classroom, and the courts to protest economic inequality, racial injustices, environmental threats, the war in Vietnam, and discrimination based on sexuality, sex, and gender. Pushing back against the social upheaval brought about by leftist activists, conservatives quickly responded with protests of their own. The dramatic upheaval of these decades continued into the 1980s and 1990s and led to unparalleled social change and political conflict that still resonates today.

Beginning in the mid-twentieth century but drawing on decades of prior activism, self-proclaimed "feminists" dreamed of, nay, demanded, an egalitarian society in which the sexes were equal both legally and socially. They devised experiments in which to test their ideas about equality and sought places to put their theories into action. Many wondered what egalitarian feminism actually looked like in practice. Naturally, as they practiced feminism in new ways, they returned to their theories and re-evaluated their ideas. Women of color, indigenous women, lesbian women, and older women in particular demanded constant re-evaluations of the ways feminists put their theory into practice.

From the 1960s on, varieties of U.S. feminism proliferated, and activists and scholars have demarcated them generally along these lines: Black feminism saw racism and gender discrimination as intricately linked (which some call "intersectionality"). Indigenous or Native American feminism made a similar argument but also argued that decolonization and indigenous sovereignty were essential parts of achieving equality. Liberal feminists wanted to achieve equality between men and women by reforming mainstream institutions and integrating women into existing structures; they are most well known for advocating for equal pay and voting rights and are often associated with the National Organization for Women (NOW). Radical feminists believed in a total overthrow of patriarchal society and the creation of completely new woman-run institutions. Cultural feminists, which some saw as a subset of radical feminists, believed that society needed a female "essence" and that the qualities women held were both unique and superior to those of men. Lesbian feminists wanted to trouble the idea that heterosexuality was the "natural" way of life by examining its roots in patriarchal institutions. Some believed in lesbian separatism, in which women removed themselves from mainstream society and lived and worked together in a community setting. In many cases, activists themselves did not subscribe to any particular label other than "feminist" (and some did not even use that one). Most fell into more than one camp; there were Native American radical feminists, White lesbian women who subscribed to liberal feminism, Black cultural feminists, and so forth. Sometimes the differences between camps have been exaggerated, and the differences *within* a subset of feminism may have even been more significant.[2]

Many other modes of feminism existed, and they have continued to evolve and emerge, but these are the ones I see as most relevant to the self-help movement. Self-help borrowed from many strains of feminism, *and* it helped develop feminist thought. For example, self-help activists contributed to radical and cultural feminism by creating spaces for people with female bodies. They saw the female body and its capabilities as special and powerful and emphasized its uniqueness. African American and Native self-help activists forced other feminists to reconsider their definition of reproductive rights. Alongside liberal feminists, self-help activists worked to change laws and effect change by reforming existing patriarchal systems (such as mainstream medicine). In fact, the self-help movement frequently put various strains of feminism in conversation with each other, forcing each camp to reckon with the others. Further, the self-help movement forced various camps to reflect on how they defined themselves and what their own priorities and strategies were. Because self-help and feminism developed alongside each other, an examination of the self-help movement complicates and expands upon our view of feminism. This book may serve as a small taste of many of the key debates in the feminist movement.

In addition, self-help was connected to the women's health and pro-choice movements. The women's health movement included feminist activists and other healthcare providers, all of whom were interested in improving the provision of healthcare for women in the late twentieth century. Sometimes it is impossible to see the lines between self-help and this movement; at other times, they are more clear. The pro-choice or abortion rights movement included feminists, but also doctors, clergy, and lawmakers. This group sometimes overlapped with the women's health movement. To some extent, the book also explores how self-help complicated each of these movements as well. Other able scholars have conducted wonderful studies of these movements, but I touch on them where appropriate.[3]

Self-help was one of the countless ways that feminists put theory into action. This book traces the evolution of feminist self-help from its emergence as a movement in the late 1960s to the 1990s. Self-help activists helped to revolutionize women's healthcare by creating an entire system of alternative healthcare options. Some women practiced gynecological healthcare procedures, including abortions and donor insemination, in their own homes. Others, especially middle-class White women, opened clinics to make this system of care available to a wider array of women. Self-help activists both cooperated with and fought against medical providers to improve mainstream care for women. Women of color and indigenous women founded local and national organizations and used self-help to address the myriad ways racism and colonialism affected their health. As more women learned about these alternative do-it-yourself care options through media attention, written texts, and videos, the movement diversified and grew, new self-help activists developed new theories, and the meaning and practice of "self-help" changed as a result.

Those who have heard of feminist self-help are likely familiar with this "origins story": In April 1971, at a feminist gathering in the back of the Everywoman's Bookstore near Los Angeles, Carol Downer, an activist who had recently become interested in women's liberation and abortion (which was illegal until 1973), sat on a table, pulled up her skirt, and showed a group of mostly White, middle-class women how she could view her own cervix (the opening into her uterus) using a plastic speculum, a mirror, and a flashlight. The group also discussed teaching themselves to perform abortions using a suction method. These women began meeting regularly to practice cervical self-examination in small gatherings they called "self-help groups." One group member, Lorraine Rothman, created the Del-Em, a device used to remove the contents of the uterus during menstruation or early pregnancy. The group named the procedure "menstrual extraction." Over the next year, as Downer and Rothman toured the United States demonstrating both self-exam and menstrual extraction, feminist self-help groups emerged around the nation. "My God . . . I'd follow her anywhere," one self-help activist recalled thinking the first time she saw Downer climb lithely onto a table with no pants and demonstrate self-exam.[4]

Yet self-help was much, much more than this story. It was more than cervical self-exam, more than Downer or Rothman. Indeed, it was even more than the Del-Em, menstrual extraction, or abortion. Self-help was an entire movement of women taking control of their own bodies and minds. Self-help was education, prevention, treatment, peer power, protest, and politics. Self-help was a redefinition of healthcare. For some women, self-help was the difference in life and death.

Divisions

The first chapter of this book explores how gynecological self-help activism began to gather steam in the late 1960s, especially among middle-class White women, and follows feminist activists seeking to spread ideas about self-help around the nation in the early 1970s. During this time, self-help activists focused their efforts largely on cervical self-exam and menstrual extraction, believing that control over reproduction was the key to liberation. Early self-help activists faced opposition from other feminist, women's health, and reproductive rights activists. Menstrual extraction in particular provoked great controversy. At the heart of many debates among feminists was the question, Should feminist women create their own institutions or work to change existing ones? I call this debate "separate or infiltrate?" Indeed, this question was often at the heart of the divide between liberal and radical feminists. The first chapter introduces readers to this question and begins to explore how self-help activists wrestled with this key feminist debate.

Because of its roots in underground abortion, one might assume that gynecological self-help disappeared after *Roe v. Wade* legalized abortion in 1973; in fact, the decision helped accelerate its dissemination and diversify its uses. Chapter 2 explores how, in the 1970s, feminists responded to the *Roe* decision by opening dozens of woman-controlled feminist clinics to provide abortions and use self-help to develop reproductive healthcare services.[5] These clinics challenged the medicalized healthcare model by employing large numbers of staff who lacked formal medical training and by directly providing clients with knowledge about their bodies. In these woman-controlled clinics, thousands of clients learned and practiced self-help techniques, and many went on to form their own groups. Clinics operated at the nexus of the separation versus infiltration debate. Woman-controlled clinics were "alternative" healthcare institutions that employed mostly laywomen (a radical practice) and empowered clients with knowledge about their bodies. At the same time, these clinics had to operate within the confines of laws that restricted medical practice. For example, laws typically required that they hire doctors to perform abortions, instead of allowing laywomen to do them, so most feminist clinics had to employ physicians.

The second chapter also explores other debates central to the feminist movement. For example, many woman-controlled clinics began as an exercise in collectivism, or sharing control democratically among a group of invested parties, a concept near and dear to the hearts of many 1970s feminists. Clinics had varying degrees of success with this model, particularly because they were simultaneously wrestling with internal conflicts over race, class, and sexuality.

Meanwhile, activists developed a range of controversial strategies that took self-help beyond clinic walls; their activities in the 1970s and early 1980s are the subject of chapters 3 and 4. Some women formed groups to investigate and curb what they believed were harmful activities of healthcare providers, including local hospitals, other clinics, and Planned Parenthood. Other women formed "advanced" self-help groups and further explored controlling their reproduction by experimenting with new forms of birth control, donor insemination, and nonmedical menopause interventions. These chapters ask how gynecological self-help activists dealt with questions such as, To what extent should women use their own bodies to challenge patriarchal institutions? Should feminists withdraw their support from reproductive rights organizations whose goals and strategies do not line up precisely with their own? How should feminists react when their own small organizations grow so large that some measure of "male" bureaucracy is necessary?

While White women tended to focus on self-help gynecology, women of color and indigenous women expanded the definition of self-help to include examination of all aspects of their health, which they understood to be shaped by the interlocking oppressions of racism, classism, sexism, and heterosexism. In the 1980s, one group of African American women developed "psychological self-help" to dialogue about high rates of poverty, low self-esteem, and stress. Another used elements of psychological self-help and gynecological self-help to help women living with HIV/AIDS cope with their disease and the accompanying social stigma. Native American women in South Dakota created a philosophy of "holistic" self-help that merged traditional and modern methods to confront fetal alcohol syndrome and related community health issues. Chapter 5 details how women of color and indigenous women sought ways to tackle issues most important to their communities and created self-help methods that considered women's whole bodies and minds, not just their reproduction. This chapter furthers our emerging understanding of how women of color and indigenous women shaped the course of both feminism and self-help, forcing White activists to consider a wider range of women's issues.

In the late 1980s and early 1990s, just as self-help activism was extending its reach beyond gynecology, a growing conservative backlash against feminism and abortion rights led many activists to refocus their efforts on ensuring women's access to abortion. Chapter 6 explores how, in 1988, with anti-abortion groups and state and federal governments increasingly restricting the availability and legality of abortion, a group of self-help activists returned to menstrual extraction and began a push to disseminate information about it across the nation. They flaunted this technique as an early abortion method to remind the government and the public that making abortion illegal would not make it disappear. Complicating accounts of the reproductive rights movement that have portrayed this period as one of retrenchment, self-help activists taught menstrual extraction to groups of women around the United States in order to draw public attention to the growing threats to abortion rights. The holistic self-help focus often promoted by Black and Native American self-help activists during roughly the same time period was not present in this campaign, as menstrual extraction advocates believed that the urgency of the situation dictated that they put all of their eggs in the abortion basket. Still seeking to answer the "separate or infiltrate" question, self-help activists found that fear that *Roe v. Wade* would be overturned led many ordinary women to support separation. Thousands of women around the nation rallied to let the government and the American public know that women would go "underground" if they lost their right to legal abortion.

Boundaries

The self-help movement ultimately drew women from many walks of life. In fact, it is not always easy to determine which women were part of the movement, but in general, most self-help activists shared a few traits. First, they believed that mainstream medicine disempowered women. Second, they attempted to empower themselves and other women through demystification—developing an understanding of their own bodies and minds (usually in groups together). They saw this understanding as crucial to attaining autonomy and control. Some groups learned how their physical bodies functioned and taught each other basic medical procedures. Others dissected their innermost thoughts and feelings, searching for internalized racism and sexism that caused them negative emotions or manifested physically. Third, they were in constant debate with one another over the possibilities, meanings, and principles of self-help. Many argued over the extent to which self-help activists should attempt to work with mainstream medical institutions or create their own separate institutions. They debated the merits of using their energies toward disseminating information about self-help to other women. They also communicated a range of opinions about whether self-help activities should focus on gynecology, especially self-exam and menstrual extraction, or on a more holistic view of health. Finally, these activists saw self-help as central to feminism; it was a way to achieve many of the larger goals of the feminist movement. They believed that self-help could give women much of what they were fighting for—autonomy over their own bodies, minds, health, and lives. They saw self-help as a way to "do" feminism." Activists made explicit connections between their personal self-help efforts and a larger political purpose. They argued that only through controlling the terms of their own reproduction, mental and physical health, and healthcare could women achieve true equality and autonomy.[6]

Much of the literature on the women's health movement has focused on childbirth, especially midwifery and home birth. Scholarship about natural childbirth, medical interventions in childbirth, and the Lamaze technique offers an important framework for this project, demonstrating the myriad ways women have taken charge of their own birth experiences. Some of the self-help activists discussed in this book experimented with home birth, but their records of these experiments are few and far between. Many women found the self-help movement out of frustrations with their own birth experience. A close examination of the relationship between their activities and the home birth and midwifery movements is beyond the scope of this study but offers fertile ground for future scholarship.[7]

Another popular topic among scholars of the women's health movement is the seminal *Our Bodies Ourselves*.[8] In 1969, twelve women at a women's liberation conference in Boston decided to research and compile information on women's bodies and health. They published their work as an accessible booklet called *Women and Their Bodies: A Course by and for Women.* The group formally incorporated as the Boston Women's Health Book Collective and changed the name of the book to *Our Bodies, Ourselves (OBOS)* in the early 1970s. Ordinary women made contributions to each new, expanded edition of the book, and *OBOS*, through its many international iterations, became what feminist scholar Kathy Davis calls, "a global feminist project of knowledge." Millions of copies of *OBOS*, in dozens of languages, continued to sell all over the world over the next half-century.[9] Hundreds of other books designed to give women basic information about their bodies and health emerged in the wake of *OBOS*; many included differentiated material for women across a spectrum of ages, races, ethnicities, abilities, and sexualities. Some self-help practitioners studied and shared the book and were often in dialogue with its authors; some contributed sections to new editions. I leave most discussion of the far-reaching effects of *OBOS* to other able scholars but touch on it where appropriate.

This is not a comprehensive history of the self-help movement. Such a history would be impossible because of the grassroots nature of both self-help and feminism. Instead, this book traces projects that self-consciously denoted themselves as "self-help," a label I believe they used strategically. Early in the 1970s, self-help became one of the defining features of the women's health movement, and the term became associated with gynecology, self-exam, menstrual extraction, and abortion. Yet the women of color and indigenous self-help activists who moved beyond these practices and even beyond gynecology purposefully employed the term. To do so was a radical act. It declared that women's health meant more than gynecology, that to take self-help seriously meant looking beyond the cervix, to the whole woman. To understand and take women's health and reproduction seriously, one had to look at a woman as an entire being, a *raced* being.

I mean to simultaneously honor the contributions of early gynecological self-help practitioners, including Carol Downer, and also to broaden our understanding of self-help to include the other women who made self-help a movement of massive proportions. In part, I borrow my perspective on Downer as leader from historian Stephanie Gilmore's terrific examination of NOW's first president, Betty Friedan: "Love her or hate her, Friedan helped change the lives of millions of women and men. . . . But allowing her to stand for the whole of NOW's history . . . ignores the realities of the women who comprised the women's movement."[10] The same holds true for Downer. Long viewed as the "mother" of self-help, Downer did indeed contribute to a movement that continues to affect women's healthcare today. So too did the thousands of other feminist activists who questioned, expanded, and redefined self-help throughout the second half of the twentieth century and beyond. Further, I aim to expand history's view of Downer and her close associates; they were more than the "inventors" of self-exam. Many of these "original" self-help activists, responding to the growing parameters of self-help, took part in self-help activism that went well "beyond the speculum."[11]

Antecedents

For centuries, women have shared information about health and healing with one another and have sought to control their bodies and provide healthcare for their communities. From the seventeenth century through the nineteenth, slaveholders forced enslaved women to bear children to increase their labor force, and many tried to suppress traditional knowledge of birth control and abortion. Enslaved women often carried the weight of healing for the Black community and sometimes for Whites as well. They grew medicinal herbs, "caught" babies, tended the sick, and prepared the dead for burial.[12] Similarly, both before and after European contact, Native American women often assumed the routine care of their sick family members, and some cared for their entire community as midwives, pharmacists, diagnosticians, healers, and surgeons. In the name of eugenic "science," in the twentieth century, the U.S. government forced thousands of Native American, Black, Latino, immigrant, imprisoned, disabled, and indigent men and women to undergo sterilization or abortion without their knowledge or consent. Language barriers, fear of deportation, and insurance restrictions have meant that many Asian American, Latina, and immigrant women were unable to rely on institutional medicine. Women of color and poor women in the late twentieth century experienced disproportionately high rates of illness, largely as a result of lack of access to the medical system. Many U.S. hospitals admit only patients referred by a doctor, and many doctors did not accept Medicaid. Federal budget cuts to inner-city and rural health centers, food stamps, WIC (Special Supplemental Nutrition Program for Women, Infants, and Children), and school lunch programs furthered systemic health problems in communities of color. Women in these communities often turned to each other for healthcare and family planning when they could not find culturally competent health services.[13]

Women have always found ways to regulate the timing of their pregnancies, whether it was legal to do so or not. In the late nineteenth and early twentieth centuries, a contraceptive black market raged in the United States, and men and women engaged in the illicit trade of a wide variety of prophylactic devices ranging from leftover sausage casings to watch springs. Before *Roe v. Wade* legalized abortion in 1973, women were so adept at finding ways to terminate their pregnancies, usually through "back-alley" providers, referrals, and underground networks, that the numbers of abortions before and after *Roe* remained essentially constant.[14]

While these histories offer evidence of important precedents to the self-help movement, self-help activism in the late twentieth century was distinct from women's earlier efforts to pass down their health wisdom, provide healthcare for their communities, and control their bodies and reproduction. Self-help activists were self-consciously political; they enacted their feminism by practicing healthcare on their own bodies and often encouraging other women to do the same. They created a national movement of women collectively voicing a feminist critique of, and offering alternatives to, mainstream medicine.

Though self-help later came to encompass much more than abortion or even gynecology, the movement's rise was deeply interlaced with early abortion rights activism. The ability to control the timing of childbirth is well known as the heart of much of middle-class White feminism. Later chapters discuss how women of color and indigenous women in particular have long seen abortion as only one of many ways for women to control their bodies and reproduction, whereas many, though certainly not all, White feminists saw abortion as the *key* strategy for securing women's empowerment. For decades, women of color and indigenous women have insisted that White feminists should expand their focus, arguing that many "mainstream" feminist issues were not actually the issues most important to all women. Scholars have begun to document how women of color and indigenous women broadened the reproductive health agenda and popularized the concept of "reproductive justice."[15] Reproductive justice advocates recognized that historically, the "choice" to use birth control or have an abortion was not enough to guarantee a woman control over her reproduction. They argued that rather than choice, women needed *access* both to culturally appropriate medical care that included abortion and to social supports that enabled them to have and raise healthy children. Similar dynamics took shape among self-help activists. While White feminists focused largely on self-help gynecology, women of color included examination of many aspects of their health, especially those perpetuated by the interlocking oppressions of racism, classism, sexism, and heterosexism. By exploring how Black and indigenous women used self-help to deal with issues such as low self-esteem, high blood pressure, stress, HIV/AIDS, fetal alcohol syndrome, and alcoholism, this book shows how they expanded the movement and made its focus more holistic.

While many scholars note that self-help practices played a critical role in the women's health and reproductive rights and justice movements, this book is the first historical study to show how these practices evolved, diversified, and persisted throughout the late twentieth century.[16] Self-help activists created their own unique strand of theory and activism that changed over time while both clashing with and complementing other feminist health efforts. Women created a self-help movement that was far more extensive, interactive, and contested than scholars have previously recognized.

1

Enacting Feminism

The Origins of Gynecological Self-Help

> Letting us look at ourselves is like giving guns to the slaves—it gives us control over our own bodies.
> —Unknown self-help group participant

Gynecological self-help activists put nascent feminist theories about bodily autonomy into action. The roots of this process began with women active in the broader feminist movement. Early self-help groups that consisted largely of White, middle-class participants mirrored the focus of White feminist and women's health activism in their emphasis on reproductive rights, particularly abortion. Gynecological self-help activism borrowed from and expanded upon strategies developed in feminist consciousness-raising groups and abortion rights activism.

Gynecological self-help was contested terrain from its earliest iterations. Fed up with the way the state and the male medical establishment held authority over their health, self-help activists sought ways to control not only their own bodies, but also the messages and procedures associated with their health. They faced opposition from all corners, including other feminist organizations, reproductive rights advocates, abortion providers, and members of the medical community. Many such groups believed that self-help could be detrimental to women's health or to the reproductive rights movement. Self-help activists also faced internal opposition, as different camps clashed over what constituted self-help and what methods were most effective for helping women gain autonomy over their own bodies. In particular, some self-help activists believed that self-examination and menstrual extraction were the keys to women's self-sovereignty. Others believed that, while one or both of these techniques were interesting and important, they were not the zenith of women's empowerment. In spite of the contentious nature of self-help, the movement created a space and a process for a grand feminist experiment in women's healthcare provision. What began in the back room of a local bookstore as a small-scale attempt at controlling abortion soon blossomed into a national movement with interests well beyond abortion.

Women Seek Control of Abortion before *Roe v. Wade*

Until around 1880, abortions were legal in the United States until "quickening," the time when a woman could first feel the fetus moving. In general, abortions were the purview of midwives or homeopaths, not professionally trained physicians. In the mid-1800s, out of a "desire to win professional power, control medical practice, and restrict their competitors," the fledgling American Medical Association began pushing to make abortion illegal. When abortions became illegal in the 1880s, women continued to find them illegally, especially from midwives and sympathetic doctors or by traveling to places where abortion was legal. In fact, women were so successful at finding abortions during the time when it was criminalized in the United States that there were no significant differences between the numbers of abortions performed before and after *Roe*.[1]

In the midcentury United States, doctors, lawyers, clergy, and women's groups advocated for the repeal of abortion restrictions. Those who saw the horrors of botched abortions advocated for legal reform. Lawyers brought suits to help women and doctors on the hook for obtaining and providing abortions. Hundreds of clergy members and feminist groups set up underground referral networks to help women find ways to terminate their pregnancies.

While some feminist groups focused on legislation and referrals, others, such as the California-based "Army of Three," also shared information about abortion techniques with ordinary women. The Army of Three (Patricia Maginnis, Lana Clarke Phelan, and Rowena Gurner) is most famous for advocating the complete repeal of abortion laws in the United States beginning in 1959. They argued that decisions about abortion should be left to women, not to politicians and doctors. They also created a list of referrals to men and women willing to provide abortions, mostly in Mexico, and handed out thousands of copies.

The Army of Three was the first well-known activist group to flaunt the fact that women could do abortions for themselves if necessary. They began holding classes in which they helped women write letters to politicians asking for the repeal of abortion laws, discussed obtaining an illegal abortion, and learned about sterile procedures and how to use the "digital method," in which a woman inserted her finger into the opening of her uterus until she aborted. They even created and sold $2 "abortion kits" containing everything a woman would need to sterilize her bathroom and hands before using the digital method. The Army of Three warned that do-it-yourself methods were dangerous and could cost a woman a lot of money in medical procedures. They encouraged such methods only as a last resort.

Maginnis, Phelan, and Gurner advertised their classes and made sure that local police knew about them; they hoped that an arrest might lead to a court case in which they could fight for the repeal of abortion laws. In 1969, Phelan and Maginnis also published *The Abortion Handbook for Responsible Women*. In addition to information about where to get an illegal abortion, they included very detailed information on how a woman could fake a hemorrhage in order to convince a hospital that she needed an abortion. The little book sold over 50,000 copies. The three women were arrested in San Mateo County, California, for holding classes and selling the kits.[2]

Meanwhile, in Chicago, another group of women demonstrated a different way that women could take control of abortion. The Abortion Counseling Service of Women's Liberation, usually called the Jane Collective or simply Jane, was a group of women who began making abortion referrals to underground providers starting in 1969. Their goal was to help women find safe and affordable abortions. The Janes soon grew frustrated at the cost of abortions and the quality of care many of the local underground providers offered. They also learned that the man they sent most of their referrals to was not actually a licensed physician. Several members began to wonder if they too could learn to provide abortions and soon discovered that the procedure was quite simple. From 1968 to 1972, the Janes provided over 11,000 abortions to women in the Chicago area.[3]

Jane strove to provide "feminist" abortions by encouraging women to learn about their own bodies as part of their procedures. When a woman came to them for an abortion, she also left with copies of *Our Bodies, Ourselves*, *The Birth Control Handbook*, and *The VD Handbook* so that she could arm herself with as much knowledge about her body as possible. The Janes believed that they were acting to help their "sisters" and saw the women receiving abortions as "partners in the crime of demanding the freedom to control our own bodies and our own childbearing."[4] They did not teach women to perform abortions for themselves but did sometimes recruit members from among women who had used their services. Unlike the Army of Three, publicity was not their goal.

Harvey Karman Develops the Flexible Cannula

As feminist groups worked to give women control over abortions, a University of California student named Harvey Karman began exploring technology that would make abortions safer and simpler. Karman became interested in abortion technology in the 1950s while conducting research on the emotional aspects of therapeutic abortion. After learning about one UCLA student who committed suicide when she could not obtain an abortion and a second who died of a botched abortion, he began working to help women find illegal abortions in Mexico. While doing this work, Karman encountered many women who were unable to afford to travel to Mexico and others who were suffering because of the poor care they received there. He decided to learn how to perform abortions himself and began offering them illegally. One acquaintance, Dr. Phillip Darney, chief of gynecology and obstetrics at San Francisco General Hospital, said that Karman's goal was to "make it possible for women to safely do their own abortions using the simplest possible equipment."[5]

By the time Karman began learning to do abortions, many abortion providers around the country were already familiar with a variety of suction methods. Suction abortions were an alternative to the more common dilation and curettage (D&C) method, in which a provider dilated a woman's cervix and then scraped out the contents of her uterus with a spoon-like instrument. Suction abortion had become popular in Russia and China in the early twentieth century and then began slowly spreading to the United States. However, it was Karman's reliance on the "Karman cannula" that launched suction abortion into the U.S. mainstream and made it possible for laypersons (including feminist self-help activists) to begin experimenting with the procedure. Karman claimed that he developed this device while serving a prison sentence for providing an illegal abortion in California in the 1960s. Earlier cannulas were either made of solid metal, which meant that they were more likely to puncture the lining of a woman's uterus, or were so large that providers had to dilate a woman's cervix before using them, which typically required a local anesthetic. These earlier versions of the cannula were not disposable and had to be sterilized between each use. The cannula Karman used was thin, flexible, and disposable, which eliminated many of the risks and challenges of suction abortion. Self-help activists experimenting with menstrual extraction in the early 1970s would rely heavily on this technology.[6]

After his release, Karman continued experimenting with the flexible cannula, and with the help of medical writer and women's health activist Merle Goldberg, he developed a method of early suction abortion. Using a vacuum syringe and the flexible cannula, one could manually extract the contents of the uterus during the first few weeks after a missed period. The procedure was so fast compared to other contemporary methods of abortion that some began to call it the "lunch-hour abortion." Other names included uterine aspiration, manual vacuum aspiration, menstrual induction, and, most commonly, menstrual regulation.[7] A few of his physician friends gave him fetal tissue that they had removed while performing abortions. Karman practiced suctioning the tissue through cannulas of different sizes and soon discovered that he could aspirate fetal tissue up to twelve weeks of development with his small cannula. Convinced that this technology was going to revolutionize abortion procedures around the world, Karman even created a television commercial advertising free suction abortions. He was arrested again, and after his release from prison, Karman began to refer to himself as a doctor (he held a bachelor's degree in theater and a master's in psychology), a habit that would later cause great friction between him and the self-help community. Nonetheless, the medical community began using the "Karman cannula" regularly to provide suction abortions.[8]

Consciousness-Raising as a Precursor to Self-Help

Recalling a feminist meeting at the Cleveland Women's Liberation Center, health activist and author Barbara Ehrenreich wrote, "I remember the relief in the room when a group of women . . . discovered that every one of us had been told, at one time or another, that her uterus was undersized, misshapen, or misplaced. How could every woman's body be somehow abnormal and pathological?"[9] What Ehrenreich described was not atypical; in newly formed feminist groups beginning in the 1960s, women took turns discussing their personal experiences with healthcare, abortion, domestic violence, childbearing, sex, and motherhood. Hearing the similarities in each other's stories validated the women's experiences and helped the group understand that their personal problems were often the result of systemic oppression. Especially popular among young, middle-class, White women, this practice became known as consciousness-raising (CR). One participant said that CR was "a safe place for women to come together and talk about what was true for them."[10] Dialoguing about their previous health experiences became particularly popular in CR groups; many women shared their frustration with the typical gynecological exam in which a doctor focused on examining a woman's body and had little interest in hearing a patient's thoughts about her health.[11] In many cases, discovering that other women had had the same experiences and feelings created a bond of sisterhood and empowered women to take action to remedy their situations. Many were fed up with state control over abortion and birth control and with male-dominated medicine in general. Though they frequently discussed the specific complaints that were the result of having female bodies, many feminist CR groups began celebrating their bodies, exalting the wonders of the female reproductive system. Having a vagina, a cervix, a uterus, and breasts, as well as a body that could carry, birth, and nourish babies, was special, worthy of honoring. It even meant that some CR participants felt that they belonged to a kind of exclusive club. Though they celebrated differences among women's bodies, having a female body was the ticket into this club. The female body itself was a source of inquiry and study.

Because so many feminists' grievances stemmed from their existence within anatomically female bodies, gynecological self-help made sense as the next step after CR. Early 1970s self-help practitioners would focus mainly on gynecology as the key to women's ability to control their own bodies. Learning how to treat minor infections, conduct their own Pap smears, and even perform abortions meant liberation from the male-dominated medical system. The more feminists learned about their bodies and how many procedures they could do for themselves, the angrier they became about male-dominated women's healthcare.

Cervical Self-Examination Emerges

In 1969, burgeoning activist Carol Downer joined a Los Angeles NOW chapter and began learning about abortion and its history from Army of Three member Lana Phelan. In 1970, members of the Los Angeles feminist community, including the local NOW chapter, supported Harvey Karman and his colleague, John Gwynn, when they opened an illegal abortion clinic. Downer and her friends referred women to Karman and Gwynn for illegal abortions but soon began to feel "dissatisfied with the back-alley atmosphere of the clinic."[12] Though Karman and Gwynn were working to make abortion more available, this loosely organized group of feminists also decided that Karman and Gwynn were, in Downer's words, "male chauvinist pigs" because of the patronizing and disrespectful ways they spoke to women.[13] Downer recalled one telling incident when Gwynn, annoyed at her input, covered her mouth with a piece of tape and told her to be quiet.[14] She and a small group of other women began contemplating opening their own underground, woman-controlled abortion clinic. One woman who worked closely with Karman on abortion procedures told Downer and her friends that "abortion wasn't as difficult as it was made out to be" and suggested that they could learn to perform abortions on their own.[15] Karman agreed to let them observe his methods at the clinic. Remembering these events, Downer was careful to say that Karman did not *teach* them how to do abortions; he merely allowed them to observe. "He didn't give us a minute of his time, really, but he did allow us to hang out." Downer was particularly interested in the less-traumatic suction method Karman employed and was fascinated to see just how simple the procedure was.[16]

Also in Karman and Gwynn's illegal clinic, observing an IUD insertion, Downer saw a woman's cervix for the first time.[17] "I was absolutely amazed . . . it was so close! . . . My knees buckled. I was that awestruck." She took a plastic speculum from the clinic, went home, and tried it for herself. Lying in her bed, she used the plastic speculum, a flashlight, and a mirror to conduct a self-examination. Seeing her own cervix so close and accessible made Downer begin to feel confident that she and other laywomen could easily learn to perform abortions. "I had read *The Abortion Handbook* [by the Army of Three] and realized that if women just had some basic information about their bodies they . . . wouldn't have to depend on back-alley abortionists," she recalled.[18]

Around the same time, police raided Karman and Gwynn's illegal clinic, and many members of the feminist community picketed to support the two men and the three women staff members who were arrested. When Karman and Gwynn went on trial, Downer and her group hated that the pro-choice media focused more on the heroic and charismatic Karman and Gwynn than on a woman's right to an abortion or on the women who were also arrested.[19] Friction grew between the male abortion providers and the women who supported them. Downer recalled that this growing hostility only strengthened her group's resolve to take abortion into their own hands.[20]

On April 7, 1971, Downer and about thirty other women met in the back of the Everywoman's Bookstore in Venice, California, to discuss opening their own abortion clinic. Most of the attendees had answered an "enigmatic" ad in a feminist newspaper calling for women who were interested in underground abortion. The story of what happened in this meeting soon became the stuff of feminist legend.[21]

When it was her turn to talk, Downer showed the other women the suction device that Karman used to perform abortions in his clinic. It was clear to her that they were terrified. "They were in agony . . . the whole subject was scary to them. I could see that until I demystified this for them, they were going to keep on thinking that abortion was this thing that you mostly would die of." Downer decided to show the other women how easily she could do a self-exam and how accessible the cervix was. She cleared off a desk, climbed onto it, hitched up her long skirt (she was not wearing underwear), and inserted a speculum into her vagina. At first the rest of the women stood back, and Downer began to worry. "I thought, oh, they're gonna think I'm an exhibitionist!"[22] She remembered thinking that if any woman had so much as snickered or looked offended, she would have stopped immediately.[23] Instead, the other women in the room slowly began to crowd in close to see her cervix and share their excitement.[24] Eager to see their own cervixes, several other women in the group took a turn on the table doing self-exam.[25]

Many feminists believe that self-help was "born" that day in the Everywoman's Bookstore. Maybe it was. Being able to examine their own bodies in this fashion opened up whole realms of possibilities for this group of feminists. They wondered, If the cervix was so accessible, but no woman in the group had ever examined hers before, what else did she not know about her body? What else could women learn about their anatomy and reproduction if they tried? Most importantly, how could cervical self-exam allow a woman increased control over her own health? Regardless of whether self-help was "born" that day or not, ultimately the movement would grow so large, take on so many forms, look so many ways, and go so far beyond self-exam that many of the women in the Everywoman's Bookstore that day would not recognize it. Though this moment was revolutionary, the revolution did not end there.

After this meeting, several of the women who had been in the bookstore began gathering on a regular basis for gynecological "self-help groups." They procured plastic speculums and met in each other's homes or in the back rooms of feminist businesses to take turns doing cervical self-examination. They also taught themselves to perform uterine size checks on each other using a bimanual exam, did breast exams, and dialogued about their gynecological health. By examining each other's bodies on a regular basis, these self-help groups furthered their understanding of how women's bodies varied.[26] These self-help groups were the cornerstone of a feminist experiment in putting theory into action. Self-help activists saw their actions as a way to *do* something about the abysmal state of women's healthcare and to take concrete steps toward controlling their own reproduction.

Gynecological self-help spread like wildfire, first in the Los Angeles area, then throughout California and beyond. Some of the women from the original group formed spin-off groups in their own neighborhoods and communities. Many new self-help groups began as groups of friends, while others formed as groups of women responded to ads and flyers in feminist publications and businesses.[27] Dozens of women, from both the original group and spin-offs, demonstrated self-examination for other women's groups. Inspired by what they were learning, some groups began to monitor their menstrual cycles and keep careful calendars charting their basal body temperature. Others kept journals describing the quality of their vaginal secretions. A few donned white lab coats, bought urine pregnancy tests at a medical supply store, and then practiced using them. (At the time, even these simple tests were administered only in a doctor's office.) Some groups acquired microscopes to closely examine secretions, discharges, and menstrual blood. The movement had begun.[28]

The West Coast Sisters

After the meeting in the Everywoman's Bookstore, Downer and a core group of about a dozen other women met to do self-help on a regular basis and started writing about their experiences. This group sometimes called themselves the West Coast Sisters.[29] Downer, Lorraine Rothman, and Colleen Wilson were almost always part of the group, and other women came and went. The West Coast Sisters began meeting in the Los Angeles Women's Center and later founded the Feminist Women's Health Center (FWHC), where they offered self-help presentations and hosted self-help groups for the community, always emphasizing self-exam as the key to women's bodily autonomy.[30]

Because the West Coast Sisters were so prolific, their activities are more well-known than those of most other women who practiced gynecological self-help. They disseminated the story of Downer demonstrating self-exam in the Everywoman's Bookstore, sharing it with other feminists as a kind of origin myth, the genesis of the self-help movement. They also emphasized self-exam as the centerpiece of self-help. Their frequent publications and public presentations meant that they influenced thousands of other women who were experimenting with gynecological self-help. Though the West Coast Sisters were, in many ways, the voice of the burgeoning gynecological self-help movement, many women who practiced self-help or were interested in feminism more broadly disagreed with their methods and views in public forums, especially feminist periodicals.

Gynecological self-help practitioners were particularly interested in the history of the modern version of the speculum.[31] For example, in the nineteenth century, Marion Sims, often called the father of modern gynecology, conducted a variety of experimental procedures on three slave women, Anarcha, Lucy, and Betsey. Sims devised the modern "duck-billed" speculum to aid in his experimentation. Early gynecological self-helpers were aware of this history. They saw the speculum's origins as emblematic of the myriad ways medical institutions had experimented on women without their consent. Self-help practitioners replaced the cold, metal speculum of the gynecologists' office with a cheaper, plastic version. The clear design of the plastic speculum allowed them to easily observe the walls of the vagina when they inserted it. In self-help groups, a woman always inserted her own speculum. She kept the handles upright (the opposite of the way a doctor usually inserted it) in order to maintain complete control over the instrument. Self-help practitioners saw their control over the speculum as a way to demonstrate control over their own bodies. Women could buy their very own plastic speculum for around $2.[32]

The West Coast Sisters thought of self-help as a method of feminist research. For example, they conducted a menstrual cycle study, in which nine women gathered daily for a month to compile data on a thirty-six-point chart. They took measurements of temperature, did Pap smears, gathered cervical secretions, made notes about their moods, and compiled daily photographs of their cervixes. In conducting this study, the group aimed to demystify their periods and redefine a normal period and a normal body. For instance, they discovered that it was not uncommon to have a menstrual period that was longer or shorter than four days or a cervix that tipped forward or backward.[33] They defined this research as "feminist" because they used their own bodies for experimentation rather than experimenting on someone else. Further, they hoped their work would decrease male physicians' profits from and control over women's bodies. They argued that their research was more valid and reliable than that done by doctors and pharmaceutical companies because, unlike those groups, they were not interested in profits.[34]

The West Coast Sisters argued that male doctors selfishly guarded information about women's healthcare in order to maximize their profits and maintain control over women's bodies. In a 1971 article titled "Self-Help Clinic," the West Coast Sisters sprinkled dollar signs throughout the text each time they mentioned physicians. For example, after discussing the "gold mine of information" that they found when they did self-exam, the group wrote, "No wonder that physicians have been reluctant to share the information $$$." They also emphasized that a woman could be familiar enough with her body that she could recognize when going to the doctor was necessary and then advocate for her needs while she was in the examining room.[35]

Self-Help Activists Develop the "Dirty Little Machine"

Self-exam opened up a world of possibilities; the one many gynecological self-help activists seized upon immediately was feminist control of abortion. At a time when abortions were still illegal in the United States, the West Coast Sisters argued that women should not only be able to have abortions, they should be able to perform them for each other without official medical training. Their newfound knowledge of their bodies, coupled with their acknowledgment of shared women's experiences, led them to believe that this was something they could do for themselves without the help of doctors and certainly without permission from the state. After seeing Karman's suction equipment and Downer's self-exam demonstration, Lorraine Rothman decided that she could make the suction abortion kit safer and easier for laywomen to use. Karman's device, a flexible cannula attached to a syringe, was simple and efficient, but it had two major flaws: the syringe on the device could get full and need to be emptied during the procedure, and, more seriously, the person operating it could unwittingly reverse the suction and allow air to be pumped into the uterus of the woman undergoing the extraction, potentially causing a fatal air embolism. Rothman's husband, Al, a biology professor, helped her find a one-way valve to control the direction of the airflow. Rothman also added a collection tube that led into a jar so that someone using the device would not have to stop in the middle of the procedure if the syringe got full. Rothman brought the improved suction device back to the group. They began showing it to other women's health activists and to abortion providers. One doctor referred to it as a "dirty little machine," and the group adopted the name as a joke. They soon shortened the name to DLM, and then it morphed into "Del-Em."[36]

The West Coast Sisters began practicing with the Del-Em, first by suctioning water from a glass and then on each other. They called this process "menstrual extraction" and began demonstrating it to other women's groups along with self-exam. Many of those groups began practicing it among themselves. Rothman's mechanical changes meant that a menstrual extraction required the cooperation of several women working together. One person directed the cannula into the uterus of the woman having the extraction. Another pumped the syringe. Another was in charge of keeping the woman having the extraction informed and comfortable. This was purposeful; the West Coast Sisters wanted menstrual extraction to require a group. Unlike the Army of Three, they never intended their methods as a do-it-yourself procedure that women could perform solo. Unlike the Janes, at this time, they did not want to provide services to other women. They insisted that menstrual extraction was safe only when performed in a self-help group that had been meeting for several months and had gotten very well acquainted with each other's bodies. In 1974, the West Coast Sisters wrote, "As much as we advocate every woman having a speculum in her bathroom, we do not advocate that every woman have a Del'um in her bathroom." For this group, true feminism lay in working in congress with other women. Unlike a typical abortion procedure, a woman having a menstrual extraction was the equal of the women performing one, an active participant. In fact, she might even get up from her own procedure and then help perform one for her friend.[37]

Though Rothman originally developed the Del-Em so that the group could perform early abortions more safely than they could with Karman's aspiration kit, self-help activists quickly saw the potential of this suction procedure for uses beyond abortion. Because menstrual extraction worked by removing the contents of the uterus, it could bring immediate relief from cramps and other menstrual symptoms. Using menstrual extraction, women could reduce the pain and annoyance of their periods to a few minutes instead of a few days.[38] Some women in self-help groups used it every month for this purpose.[39] In fact, in spite of the Del-Em's origins as a suction abortion device, 1970s menstrual extraction advocates typically emphasized its use as a means of controlling one's period and did not call it an abortion method. At one such presentation, a woman asked, "Isn't this really an abortion technique?" Downer replied, "No. Abortion is illegal; we deal only with period extractions. . . . We're not in the martyr business."[40]

While some pre-*Roe* groups, such as the Army of Three, flaunted their activities in order to get arrested and draw attention to reproductive rights, menstrual extraction advocates, including the West Coast Sisters, were generally uninterested in this tactic during this period.[41] Publicly, gynecological self-help activists claimed that menstrual extraction was an "extralegal" procedure, one that did not fall anywhere inside the purview of the law. Among themselves, however, some groups took precautions to avoid legal trouble. A few reported that when they met to perform a menstrual extraction, members purposefully arrived separately with the various pieces of equipment, and when they met at a woman's house, they avoided attracting attention by not all parking their cars in front of the house.[42]

Menstrual extraction practitioners intended that a group of ordinary women in a self-help group could easily put together their own Del-Em. To be a truly feminist abortion procedure, it had to be democratized, available to as many women as possible. The device consisted of a Mason jar, rubber stoppers or corks, tubing from fish tanks, a syringe, a Karman cannula, and the one-way valve. Women could assemble the kit by using objects found in their home and in a few scientific product supply centers, which existed in most major cities. Rural women had to either travel or order many of these pieces by mail from medical suppliers, and some pieces could be pricey (as much as $100 total). Putting a kit together also took time, since one had to either go to a supply center or wait for a mail order. The factors of money and time, combined with the fact that menstrual extraction was safest when performed by women very familiar with each other's bodies, meant that it was rarely an ideal solution for women urgently seeking an abortion.[43]

Menstrual extraction practitioners diligently distinguished their procedure from Karman's, claiming that his suction method, menstrual regulation, was simply an abortion procedure, while their technique was a way for women to exercise control over and learn about their bodies.[44] One group of menstrual extraction practitioners affiliated with Downer's daughter, Laura Brown, wrote, "We are well aware that men are obsessed with concern over the trite issue: Did their sperm in fact fertilize the ovum?" This group claimed that when they performed menstrual extraction, they were completely unconcerned with the possibility of a fertilized egg. Instead, they said they did menstrual extraction to reduce the annoyance of their periods or as a means of learning more about their bodies. Some women saw menstrual extraction, like self-exam, as a feminist science experiment. After a menstrual extraction, women often dumped the contents of the Del-Em into a petri dish to examine them. They sometimes put the extracted material under a microscope to learn about its contents.[45] Self-help activist Barbara Hoke recalled, "We wanted to know everything the blood could teach us. . . . We practically wanted to eat it. We did taste it and smell it and study it."[46]

Even after *Roe v. Wade* legalized abortion in 1973, laypersons performing abortions could be charged with practicing medicine without a license, so menstrual extraction practitioners continued to insist that the procedure was not an abortion. Abortion, they argued, was a procedure performed by a doctor in a medical setting. They began arguing that menstrual extraction was a "home health procedure" used to "gain control over our reproductive lives."[47]

Some women even described menstrual extraction as a method of feminist, woman-controlled birth control. An Oakland group suggested that a woman who had tried several forms of birth control and found them unsuitable would be a good candidate for monthly menstrual extractions. Referring to a hypothetical woman in this situation, they wrote: "She does not want to be pregnant. Her group meets; she and they extract her period, at which point she is not pregnant. Was she or wasn't she? Who cares? She does not: the group does not." This apathy was purposeful. These self-help activists emphasized the insignificance of fertilization to reinforce the pro-choice view that a fertilized egg was not a human being. Blurring the line between birth control and abortion furthered this argument. Some self-help activists believed menstrual extraction was "vastly superior" as a method of birth control "because it involves no disruption of our daily lives and does not need to be used when it is not necessary as is the case with the pill or IUD."[48] At first, some menstrual extraction practitioners worried about the physical effects of using the procedure. Self-help activists eagerly consumed medical journals to learn about the dangers of other types of contraception and compared their findings to their newfound knowledge about menstrual extraction. Some deduced that menstrual extraction was even safer and had fewer side effects than other methods of birth control and practiced it regularly as contraception.[49]

Disseminating Gynecological Self-Help

When the West Coast Sisters developed self-exam and menstrual extraction, they believed that these methods were the key to women's liberation, and they wanted to spread the concept far and wide immediately. Like many feminists, they were exasperated that male doctors and politicians controlled a procedure that was only for women. They saw control of abortion as the epitome of bodily autonomy, the ultimate symbol of a woman's control over her own reproduction, health, and life.

The West Coast Sisters became feminist evangelists. Through workshops and mimeographed handouts, information about self-exam and menstrual extraction spread rapidly through the feminist network in the greater Los Angeles area and then beyond. Women began calling and writing to ask the West Coast Sisters to do workshops for chapters of feminist groups and on college campuses all around California. From San Francisco to San Diego, the West Coast Sisters reclined on tables, blankets, and shag rugs demonstrating self-exam and encouraging other women to look at their own cervixes. Soon women from other states also began contacting them. Then those women began spreading information about self-help to feminists they knew as well.[50] In addition to practicing self-help in groups in each other's homes and businesses, some self-help activists began running clinics, usually out of existing local women's centers. In 1971, when it appeared that abortion was on the verge of becoming legal throughout the United States, the West Coast Sisters put aside their plans to open an illegal abortion clinic and decided to travel extensively and show women how to do self-help, especially self-exam and menstrual extraction, instead. They faced immediate and continued opposition to their promotion of self-exam and menstrual extraction.[51]

Often depicted as the bastion of liberal feminism, in the 1960s and 1970s, the National Organization for Women was the largest membership-based feminist organization in the United States. Yet, as other historians have demonstrated, local chapters of NOW were often more radical and diverse than the national organization and its leadership.[52] From its inception, the self-help movement exposed this fact. The West Coast Sisters and other new self-help activists used NOW as a vehicle for their promotion of gynecological self-help, though the national organization did not always fully support their efforts. Local NOW chapters and conferences hosted self-help presentations and groups, and as NOW expanded, so did self-help. In the summer of 1971, NOW held a conference in Los Angeles.[53] The national organization refused to put a self-exam presentation on the official schedule of events, claiming that it was too shocking, so the West Coast Sisters sent out a flyer inviting other NOW delegates to see demonstrations of the technique in their hotel rooms.[54] Downer and Rothman and the other self-help activists in attendance found themselves bombarded with requests from women interested in the procedure. Delegates from local NOW chapters lined up outside of the West Coast Sisters' hotel rooms to learn about self-exam.[55] Because of the popularity, the self-help activists held a demonstration about every half hour for most of the two days, and by the end of the weekend, over two hundred women had seen a demonstration of self-exam.[56] Each woman left with her own plastic speculum in a brown paper bag.[57] Following the convention, NOW representatives from around the nation began phoning and writing the West Coast Sisters asking them to come to their cities to discuss self-help. In the fall of 1971, loaded down with two hundred speculums and bus fare, Downer and Rothman shared their knowledge in twenty-three different cities across the United States.[58] Self-help activists also continued covertly demonstrating self-exam at NOW conferences for the next few years. For example, at the Atlanta NOW Conference in 1973, Joan Edelson gathered thirty women in her hotel room to watch a slide show about self-help on a sheet pinned to the wall.[59]

The main audience for gynecological self-help presentations in the early 1970s was middle-class White women. This was largely a function of the West Coast Sisters' growing feminist network: NOW especially (though certainly not exclusively) attracted White women.[60] Downer and Rothman also presented on college campuses and in women's centers, and their audiences there were mostly White as well. This was also a result of gynecological self-help's entanglements with abortion rights work. Activist women of color in the early 1970s were often interested in a wider spectrum of reproductive rights, including sterilization abuse and access to birth control.[61] The West Coast Sisters' contacts with the abortion rights network mostly consisted of White women who encouraged them to visit their local women's groups. Some White gynecological self-help activists were concerned that they were not reaching a racially diverse audience and assumed that the reason more women of color were not involved in self-help groups was simply because they had not heard about them. They tried holding presentations in YWCAs and neighborhood associations but still did not find much enthusiasm among women of color and poor women. Later critics of gynecological self-help pointed out that it was most useful to women who mostly experienced good health. For many women of color and poor women, long-term lack of access to the medical system often meant that they had to concentrate first on serious and life-threatening health issues before they could turn to self-help.[62] Tensions over how to address the intersections of racism and sexism caused deep divisions in the wider feminist movement of the late twentieth century, and historians have only just begun to tease out the nuances of these divisions as well as the many attempts to bridge the divide. Gynecological self-help was no exception; in fact, it was a case study in the challenges inherent in organizing in the name of "universal sisterhood."[63]

Gynecological self-help quickly found audiences among both straight and lesbian women. As one woman who saw a self-help presentation in Colorado said: "My vagina is not different from anybody else's, gay or straight. I get the same infections. The male doctor who treats my infections treats me like a woman. The need to be able to care for our own bodies is common to lesbian and 'straight' women."[64] Many lesbian women were involved in the reproductive rights movement, and some self-help activists thought that self-help might attract more gay women to feminism because of its emphasis on bodily integrity and demystification. Women's health activist Cindy Pearson also suggested that many of the lesbian women in her self-help groups had been interested in practices such as menstrual extraction simply because they might "have other women in [their lives that they] cared about who might need this."[65] Later, lesbian women also took self-help practices and expanded upon them for their own purposes, experimenting with procedures such as donor insemination, for example.

Women across the country reported being enthralled when they first learned about self-help and self-exam. For many women in the 1970s, talking about and looking at their vaginas was simply unthinkable. Breaking this taboo led many to feel reverence and awe. One woman wrote that when her consciousness-raising group "first saw their cervixes they were so dizzy with enthusiasm and delight at the sheer beauty of their bodies that it was as if each woman saw a rainbow wrapped around her cervix."[66] Lolly Hirsch of Connecticut, who, with

her daughter, Jeanne, started a newsletter called the *Monthly Extract* to disseminate information about self-help, wrote, "I felt as the Great Goddess must
have felt when she created cosmos out of chaos, and stood back to view her mar-
vel."[67] Others described a new sense of ownership over their bodies. Freelance
writer Elizabeth Campbell wrote, "The first time a woman looks into her own
vagina, she knows that what she has between her legs is no longer HIS
secret—not her doctor's, not her lover's, and not Norman Mailer's." Campbell,
like many others, felt that knowledge of their bodies imbued women with power
and authority over themselves.[68]

Confronting Challenges from Local Doctors and Government Officials

In 1972, the West Coast Sisters, now operating a small clinic where women
could come to learn about self-help (the Los Angeles Feminist Women's Health
Center), began experiencing harassment from a local doctor.[69] Outraged by
publications with titles such as "Women's Self-Help Clinic: Or What to Do
While the Physician Is on His Bread-Filled Ass,"[70] a publication describing how
to use self-help when a woman was getting "no help" from her physician, the doctor reportedly called the clinic and ordered them to "change [their] literature"
because he "didn't like the way [they] attacked gynecologists." The doctor said
he "wouldn't put up with" the clinic if they refused to change their literature.[71]
The women ignored the doctor and continued to share their views about mainstream medicine.[72] Shortly thereafter, local police raided the Los Angeles
FWHC. In the process, they unwittingly brought a great deal of media attention to gynecological self-help and helped launch it into mainstream consciousness. One doctor, three uniformed policemen, and several plainclothes
investigators confiscated four trunkloads of files, books, clothes, furniture,
medical supplies, and medical equipment from the center. According to the *Los
Angeles Sentinel*, some of the clinic inspectors "made passes" at the women who
were there at the time. The staff suspected that the doctor who had made the
threatening call several months earlier was the impetus behind the raid.[73] One
self-help activist recalled that it was "like a gynecological treasure hunt" for
the police, who had an extensive list of objects they intended to confiscate. They
seized extension cords, speculums, various types of birth control (including
IUDs, pills, and diaphragms), and Del-Ems. They also removed a pie tin, a measuring cup, and a carton of strawberry yogurt from the refrigerator. According
to rumor, one staff member exclaimed, "You can't have that! That's my lunch!"[74]
This led members of the feminist community to begin referring to the raid as
"the Great Yogurt Conspiracy." The clinic members even called the raid a "feminist rape" because they felt so violated by the forceful invasion and seizure of
their property.[75]

The police brought warrants for the arrests of West Coast Sisters Carol Downer and Colleen Wilson on charges of practicing medicine without a license. The women soon discovered that the Los Angeles police had had them under surveillance for several months. They charged Wilson with helping women fit diaphragms, for giving out birth control pills, hypodermic needles, and pregnancy tests, and for drawing blood.[76] She pled guilty on one count: practicing medicine without a license because she fit a woman with a diaphragm. The court fined her $250 and sentenced her to two years' probation. Downer protested the punishment, saying that fitting a diaphragm was just like fitting a shoe. The city also charged Downer with practicing medicine without a license because she showed a woman how to do self-cervical exam and recommended that she put yogurt in her vagina to fight a yeast infection. Downer decided to stand trial for these offenses.[77]

Women and a few men around the nation rallied to support Downer in her trial, and in the process raised awareness of the self-help movement. Some compared Downer and Wilson to suffragists and early birth control advocates such as Margaret Sanger who went to jail for women's rights.[78] The *Monthly Extract* reported that outspoken feminist congresswoman Bella Abzug believed that the trial was nothing less than a test case to determine whether women were allowed to examine their own bodies.[79] Dozens of women called and wrote to Downer and the clinic offering encouragement. Several famous personalities, including Gloria Steinem, Robin Morgan, and Dr. Benjamin Spock, publicly declared their support. The clinic reported that "support from hundreds of women came in the form of donations and affidavits stating that they had used a speculum" to perform self-exam.[80] Others demanded publicly that the state provide a definition for practicing medicine. Did this include diagnosing measles? Administering an enema for a sick child? If a person thought that applying yogurt to a cold sore on her mouth might help her condition, would she be in trouble for trying this remedy? What about self-exam? Was simply looking at one's own vagina illegal?[81] Downer asked one doctor involved in her trial whether a mother diagnosing her child's illness would qualify as practicing medicine without a license. He reportedly replied, "Well, we can't do anything about *that*."[82] Feminist anthropologist Margaret Mead told the *Los Angeles Times*, "Men began taking over obstetrics, and they invented a tool . . . to look inside women. You would call this progress, except that [when] women tried to look inside themselves, this was called practicing medicine without a license."[83]

Downer's main defense was that the statute that prohibited laypeople from "diagnosing and treating" was too vague. She argued that if the state truly enforced this law, a person could not pass a sneezing friend a tissue or bring over chicken soup for a cold.[84] Downer told the press, "Our self-help clinics are much simpler than a Red Cross first aid course. . . . If we were arrested for what we did, then most of the mothers in the nation should also be in jail."[85] Jeanne Hirsch asked, "What man would be put under police surveillance for six months for looking at his penis? What man would have to spend $20,000 and two months in court for looking at the penis of his brother?"[86]

The state's main witness, Sharon Dalton, claimed that Downer had offered to perform an abortion or insert an IUD for her. The defense proved that she had not even been at the clinic on the date that Dalton claimed they spoke, and Downer was acquitted of all charges.[87] In response to the verdict, feminist Deborah Rose said, "Women in California now have the right to examine their own and each other's bodies. . . . Amazing to me that we have to win that right."[88]

After the trial, self-help practitioners found themselves barraged with interest in the use of the plastic speculum and requests for self-help presentations. *Time*, *Newsweek*, and the *New York Times* covered the event, as did a variety of local papers.[89] Lolly and Jeanne Hirsch sent copies of the *Monthly Extract* with the headline "SOS . . . Save Our Sisters . . . Save Ourselves" to dozens of feminist activists as well as all of the presidents of local NOW chapters in the United States.[90] Self-help activists across the nation saw the trial as "a great victory for self-help and for women taking control of their bodies." The attempt to squelch self-help activities had only gained more attention for the movement and piqued more women's interest in self-help techniques.[91] Yet the increased attention on self-help meant that it slipped further from the control of the West Coast Sisters. It also exposed the movement to increased criticism as less sympathetic parties became aware of it.

Defending Gynecological Self-Help

Gynecological self-help quickly gained detractors, even among feminists. Some felt shocked that self-help presenters would literally take off their pants and expose their own bodies and appalled at the suggestion that they try it themselves. After seeing self-exam for the first time, one NOW member in Orange County said, "We shouldn't be subjected to this kind of thing," and another told the group, "If this is what NOW is about, you can count me out."[92] Other women worried that the focus on gynecological self-help would take energy away from other important efforts of the women's health movement, including legislative and judicial reform. The popular feminist newsjournal *off our backs* wrote, "Self-help alone cannot confront the medical monopoly of the AMA, ACOG, the drug companies, hospitals, insurance companies, and other corporations that control our healthcare."[93] Some worried that self-help groups would merely "take the heat off" mainstream medical institutions by serving as a place for women to air their grievances without making any actual changes to the larger medical system.[94] Journalist Ellen Frankfort asked, "What good is it to know how to recognize disease if we have a health system that remains unresponsive to prevention or to the need to provide adequate care for everyone?"[95] Criticisms such as these later led many self-help activists to direct their energy into starting woman-controlled clinics as an alternative to mainstream medical institutions. These questions mirrored the "separate or infiltrate" debate in the wider feminist movement: Is it better to create change from within an existing system or to reject that system altogether and begin anew? Some women liked the idea of using self-help and self-exam as a method of educating women but were worried that an overreliance on self-help might lead women to neglect a visit to the doctor when their conditions were beyond at-home treatment.[96] Many self-help activists argued that self-help should be used in conjunction with mainstream medicine. One New Hampshire group offered the following scenario as an example of how to use self-help to enhance a visit to the gynecologist: "A practitioner might say, 'You have a mild erosion on your cervix.' And you might respond, 'I just noticed that last month, and it hasn't changed in size or color.' To which the practitioner might reply, 'Good. It's only been there for a short time. You should watch it for a few months and if it changes, I will take extra Pap smear slides.'"[97] Other self-help activists, including the West Coast Sisters, dismissed these concerns altogether, arguing that there was no evidence that mainstream medicine provided better care than women could find in self-help groups. In response to such a criticism in the *Guardian*, West Coast Sister Collette Price asked, "Is the radical press itself so mystified by the medical establishment that it too believes only a doctor can really give good safe healthcare?"[98]

Other critics were impressed by self-exam and self-help groups but stopped short of approving of menstrual extraction. Downer and Rothman visited a group of women in Gainesville, Florida, which included Byllye Avery, who were planning to open a women's clinic that emphasized self-help.[99] In addition to their fears about the safety of menstrual extraction ("We didn't know whether you would pull off some of the lining," Avery said later), the group was philosophically opposed to the idea of removing and casting aside their menstrual periods. "Our whole approach was we were making peace with our menstrual cycle. We didn't want to get rid of it in one quick thing. We wanted to know how to live with it in harmony. . . . We were more interested in turning it into a positive experience." Referring to the West Coast Sisters who visited Gainesville, Avery recalled, "They were a lot more hard-nosed feminists than we were."[100]

The West Coast Sisters and their close affiliates had little patience for those who felt unsure about menstrual extraction, and they did not hesitate to question a woman's commitment to feminism if she was not on board with the procedure. Frankfort wrote a detailed account of seeing Downer and Rothman's self-help presentation in the early 1970s, punctuating her narrative with enthusiastic phrases like "Right on!" and professing that she felt like a blind person seeing for the first time.[101] Her enthusiasm waned, however, when she began to probe Downer and Rothman more deeply with questions about the safety of menstrual extraction, and they reportedly responded by criticizing her commitment to feminism. Frankfort was dismayed that what began as such an exciting possibility ended in conflict and "dogma." She felt that after giving such a "dazzling demonstration," the self-help practitioners shut down her questions without entertaining them at all.[102] Frankfort published her account of this meeting and her experiences with self-help in the introduction to *Vaginal Politics*, her 1972 book about the politics of women's health. The Los Angeles FWHC newsletter published a scathing review of the book, written by Dorothy Tennov, a woman who had attended the same self-help presentation as Frankfort. Tennov said that Frankfort was unable to understand the political implications of self-help and the importance of the procedure as anything other than "dangerous play" undertaken by "foolish children." She characterized Frankfort's criticisms of self-help as "fussy and irrational" and argued that *Vaginal Politics* helped to maintain the medical mystification status quo. Tennov claimed that Frankfort was the only one of fifty women present to "have missed the point."[103]

Even the Jane Collective was not completely on board with menstrual extraction. A first glance at these two groups would suggest that the members of Jane and the West Coast Sisters would have had much in common and much to learn from each other. Downer and Rothman visited Chicago and demonstrated menstrual extraction for the members of Jane. As usual, they first introduced the technique as a way of removing their period, and as one Jane recalled, "Jane members wondered why a woman would put something in her uterus and risk infection to avoid having a period." However, once the Janes gleaned that menstrual extractions were also useful as a method of abortion, they grew more interested.[104]

Tensions between the two groups grew after they observed each other at work. "We talked about what we did, and they were aghast; they talked about what they did, and we were aghast," one member of Jane recalled. For example, Downer and Rothman were disdainful of Jane's methods of sterilizing tools. Rather than using an autoclave, which was too heavy and cumbersome to carry from apartment to apartment, Jane members boiled their instruments or used cold sterilizer. One member of Jane said that she thought Jane was "doing something a little more important, serious, harder than [self-help practitioners], and it took away some of their thunder." Some of the Janes were especially concerned about Downer and Rothman's relationship with Harvey Karman. One member even later wrote that the group believed that Downer and Rothman felt "reverence" for Karman. The Janes felt that the self-help practitioners wanted to be "stars" and were interested in getting attention and accolades. After spending some time at the Los Angeles FWHC, the Jane Collective decided that menstrual extraction was not the best method for them. Jane members often performed dozens of abortions a day, and menstrual extraction took twice as long as a D&C. It is likely that many West Coast Sisters would have agreed that menstrual extraction was not appropriate for Jane. They felt that menstrual extraction was an activity that a group of dedicated women in a self-help group undertook together, not a service that women provided for each other.[105]

Like many other feminists, though they were wary of menstrual extraction, the members of Jane were excited about self-exam. They began bringing mirrors to the abortions they performed. At first, they asked their clients if they wanted to see their cervix. After a while though, when most women declined the offer, they changed tactics. They began just handing clients the mirror and saying, "Here, look at your cervix." One Jane argued that this was "self-knowledge that women needed." No evidence suggests that the West Coast Sisters were aware that Jane had instituted this new tactic. Undoubtedly, however, they would have been appalled. Being instructed to look at one's cervix on an exam table would not have held the same emancipatory power as choosing to do so oneself in a self-help group.[106] Referring to a woman who had first seen her cervix when a doctor handed her a mirror on the exam table, Downer said in an interview, "Context is everything. . . . It didn't have the same impact on her. . . . [It] doesn't have the same psychological result."[107]

Gynecological Self-Help Practitioners Clash with Harvey Karman and Jane

As thousands of women around the nation learned about self-help, the meaning and practice slipped further from the West Coast Sisters' grasp, and they felt particularly concerned about losing their grip on menstrual extraction. Though they wanted women everywhere to have knowledge of this procedure, they also wanted it to look a certain way. They wanted it to stay in women's hands and *always* be practiced as a group procedure in the context of other self-help efforts. They also wanted to keep "their" procedure out of the hands of Harvey Karman.

In 1971, shortly after Downer and Rothman toured the United States, the relationship between Karman and the West Coast Sisters began to sour in earnest. Rothman published an article on self-help in a small women's newspaper called *Everywoman* and signed it "West Coast Sisters." A few months later, *Everywoman* also published an article titled "Menstrual Extraction," signed by Peggy Grau, a person unaffiliated with the West Coast Sisters. The Grau article described menstrual extraction as a "do-it-yourself" method of suction abortion and encouraged readers to learn the procedure in case they were in need.

Readers assumed that the same women were behind both articles and inundated the West Coast Sisters with questions about "self-abortion." Many of these women also sent money for the "self-abortion kit." The West Coast Sisters were utterly dismayed. They responded to as many of these requests as possible, trying to make their stance clear: menstrual extraction was not an individual abortion technique, and "the idea of 'a kit in each women's private bathroom' is anti-sisterhood . . . anti-women's liberation," and downright dangerous. Lolly Hirsch also pointed out that only a "gymnastic genius" could give herself a menstrual extraction.[108] The West Coast Sisters also immediately wrote a response to the Grau article in a NOW newsletter, saying, "THIS ARTICLE IS NOT OURS. WE CONSIDER IT IRRESPONSIBLY WRITTEN AND DANGEROUS TO WOMEN'S HEALTH."[109]

Early in 1972, the International Planned Parenthood Federation (IPPF) sent Harvey Karman on a "mercy mission" to Bangladesh to perform experimental abortion procedures on women who had been raped by Pakistani soldiers during the Bangladeshi War of Independence. The *Los Angeles Times* published an article with a picture of Karman standing with Sir Malcolm Potts, the executive director of Planned Parenthood.[110] Self-help activists who knew Karman were furious that the article had "portray[ed him] as a hero," and they "wondered how the respectable and conservative image of Planned Parenthood fit in with such a spectacular event." Karman reportedly performed this procedure on as many as 1,500 women.[111] Self-help activists associated with the West Coast Sisters denounced Karman and Planned Parenthood for using experimental methods and for not being "accountable to the women they were treating, but to a global population plan."[112] After seeing this article, the self-help activists began looking more closely at Planned Parenthood's deeper entanglements with international population control. For example, IPPF participated in a multi-organizational effort to supply Karman's menstrual regulation device to international clinics and to collect data on its use.[113] Self-help practitioners condemned these efforts as experimental, "free-wheeling practices of . . . men who function above the laws and customs of any country while wearing the guise of humanitarianism."[114]

Later, the West Coast Sisters ran an article in the *Los Angeles Women's Liberation Newsletter* with a skull and crossbones saying, "Self-menses extraction is dangerous."[115] Though it is still unclear who wrote the Grau article, the West Coast Sisters always believed that it was Karman. They contended that he was seeking publicity for his method of suction abortion by conflating it with menstrual extraction. The Los Angeles FWHC newsletter published a huge exposé on Karman's activities and accused him of writing the Grau article under a woman's name as a ploy to gain credibility among women. They pointed out that an address that appeared in the article led to a building only a few blocks from Karman's home.[116] Karman continued to make trouble for self-help practitioners when he told the *Los Angeles Free Press* that self-help activists were doing illegal abortions; the West Coast Sisters continued to receive "frantic appeals" for abortions from women all over the country.[117] They spent months replying to the women who inquired about self-abortion and illegal abortions, distancing themselves publicly from Karman, and compiling what they called the "Karman shitpile," a "file to clarify the relationship of our feminist group, the Self-Help Clinic, and Harvey Karman, and to distinguish menstrual extraction from early abortion."[118] Rothman even applied for a patent on the Del-Em.[119] The West Coast Sisters hoped that the patent might prevent Karman and other abortion providers from continuing to use the term "menstrual extraction" to describe an early abortion suction procedure and keep "Lorraine's invention" "within the women's movement."[120]

Also in 1972, Chicago police busted the Jane Collective for providing illegal abortions and shut down their operations. At the time, Jane had nearly three hundred women scheduled for procedures. They found referrals for many of the women, but about forty posed a special problem. Their pregnancies had advanced past the point when a D&C (a typical method of providing first trimester abortions) was viable, and they could not pay to travel to places such as New York where second trimester saline abortions were legal. Desperate for a way to provide the abortions for the waiting women, Jane turned to Karman, even though they had been "wary" of him since they first met him. He agreed to perform the second-term abortions for free using an experimental "supercoil" method. In this untested method, an abortion provider inserts a plastic coil through the opening of the cervix and into the uterus and removes it twelve to twenty-four hours later.[121] Fearing police surveillance after their arrests, the Jane Collective reached out to their network outside of Chicago in search of a place for Karman to perform the abortions. Dr. Kermit Gosnell, a Philadelphia practitioner who was interested in learning about the supercoil method, agreed to let Karman and the Janes use his clinic in Philadelphia for the procedures.[122] Jane reportedly contacted all of the women scheduled for an abortion, described the experimental method, and explained that they had had no prior experience with supercoils. They "felt that if they were completely honest with each woman, and gave her every bit of info that they had, then she could make her own decision." About twenty women agreed to the procedure, and Jane chartered a bus to take them to the Philadelphia clinic where the abortions were to take place. Most of the women were young, poor, Black, and likely had no other alternative for abortions. Events spiraled downward quickly. According to Jane, Karman gave information about the riskiness of supercoils to the Philadelphia clinic doctors hosting them that he had never given to the members of Jane. Jane felt that this was because "he wanted us to be dependent on him because we were women." Karman also brought along an "entourage," including a couple who were writing his biography. This made Jane members feel as if Karman were more interested in looking like a hero than in performing safe abortions.[123] One woman turned out not to be pregnant, and another four were early enough in their pregnancies that they could have a suction abortion after all. That left fifteen women to receive supercoil abortions. Of those fifteen women, nine had complications, and several ended up in the hospital with serious infections. One woman's complications were so severe that she had to have a hysterectomy at a local hospital.[124]

In response to this catastrophe, a local group called the Philadelphia Women's Health Collective published a paper they called "The Philadelphia Story." They disseminated this paper at women's conferences over the next year.[125] Jane members strongly suspected that the West Coast Sisters and members of the Los Angeles FWHC either wrote or encouraged another group to write "The Philadelphia Story."[126] Jane member Laura Kaplan later wrote that they believed the West Coast Sisters were "using it to attack their archenemy and former ally," Karman.[127] No evidence to prove this accusation surfaced, but the Los Angeles FWHC reprinted the paper in their newsletter.[128]

"The Philadelphia Story" paper placed most of the blame for the incident on Karman, denouncing both his use of the unsafe supercoil method and the publicity Karman sought for his efforts.[129] "The Philadelphia Story" stated that the members of the women's health movement who had experience with Karman, particularly the women from the Los Angeles FWHC, believed that he was "more concerned with undermining women's control of their health care and propagating his own technology and reputation than with meeting the needs of women." The Jane Collective warned that women's health activists needed to guard against men like Karman who "employ our own rhetoric about the rigidity and professionalism of the medical establishment." The Collective believed that he was exploiting women by trying to appear "hip" and anti-mainstream medicine. "Not everyone who works outside of the medical systems is working for our best interests," the Collective warned. They brought up Karman's prior attempts to claim menstrual extraction, arguing that his actions demonstrated that Karman was a person who "had no commitment to the women's movement or to women in general, but [was] . . . committed only to increasing [his] own power, reputation, and bank account." The Collective also claimed that, during previous abortions, Karman made "sexual and sexist advances on women, literally while they were on the table." They disseminated "The Philadelphia Story" to other women's groups across the country.[130]

This incident further strained the relationship between the Janes and the West Coast Sisters. Jane members continued to believe that they had acted in the best interests of women; the West Coast Sisters continued to believe that the Janes were not doing enough to put power into women's own hands. Jane members believed that the West Coast Sisters (or whoever was really behind "The Philadelphia Story") portrayed the Janes as "dupes" and the women having abortions as "ignorant poor women of color, guinea pigs experimented on without their knowledge or consent." Kaplan recalled that "The Philadelphia Story" "smacked of racism" because of its portrayal of the women having abortions.[131]

"Letting us look at ourselves is like giving guns to the slaves—it gives us control over our own bodies," said a self-help participant from Phoenix around 1976.[132] In the decades leading up to the 1970s, typically only male doctors wielding a speculum had the knowledge and ability to view a woman's cervix. Feminist activists seized the speculum and turned their gazes inward using a flashlight and a mirror. The cervix, a physical gateway, was also a metaphorical gateway to many other sources of control over their own healthcare, including menstrual extraction and countless self-help practices that would emerge over the coming decades, all of which worked to wrest power from physicians and put it in the hands of feminist women.

2

Revolutionizing
Gynecology

Self-Help in Feminist Clinics

> If you walked in the door and wanted
> our service, you [were] going to hear
> our spiel.
> —Marion Banzhaf

Gynecological self-help activists wanted to completely revolutionize the experience women had in a typical visit to the gynecologist. They objected to the inherent power dynamics of the traditional doctor-patient relationship. Prior to the 1970s, a woman usually encountered her gynecologist (who was almost always a man) when she was reclined on an exam table with her feet in stirrups. Her pelvic exam might be painful, her doctor brusque, demanding, and patronizing. He might scold her for asking about birth control, particularly if she were unmarried. If he believed she needed a medical procedure, he would likely perform it without explaining it to her or giving her much choice in the matter. Nothing about a visit to the gynecologist was empowering—quite the contrary. In an effort to change all of that, self-help activists created a form of healthcare unlike anything else in existence: the feminist clinic. In feminist clinics (often called "feminist health centers," "feminist women's health centers," "FWHCs," or simply "clinics"), the goal was for laywomen healthworkers and clients to learn from each other. Healthworkers were expected to practice self-help in order to learn about their own bodies and help clients do the same. Instead of passively receiving examinations and treatments from a physician, women in feminist health centers taught each other the basics of gynecological care. Creating a new, hybrid kind of healthcare was not easy, especially because feminist clinics were essentially a marriage between the medical system and gynecological self-help groups.

In feminist clinics, thousands of women were exposed to self-help and even feminism for the first time when they sought routine gynecological care. Many clinic employees, especially founders, believed they had a responsibility to share the principles of self-help and women's liberation. Whereas the West Coast Sisters had acted as traveling evangelists in locations such as NOW chapters and on college campuses, clinic employees could proselytize to a somewhat captive audience. In many cases, depending on their location, feminist clinics were "the only game in town" for women seeking abortions.[1]

Many obstacles threatened self-help activists' ability to put feminist theory into action in clinics. The very nature of a medical setting was contrary to the way many early practitioners envisioned gynecological self-help. In order to operate legally, clinics had to follow many of the same laws and guidelines that a traditional gynecologist's office followed. In order to provide medical services, clinics struggled to find physicians willing to work in woman-controlled businesses. They also faced restrictions and legal challenges from government institutions, particularly over their use of laywoman healthworkers. After 1973, fierce competition from other abortion providers, including Planned Parenthood, who did not follow a self-help model intensified this struggle. Many clinics also had to fight to continue operating in spite of high staff turnover and internal conflict, especially over egalitarianism, race, class, and sexuality. Yet these challenges did not stop or even slow down the spread of self-help. In fact, the movement thrived on these struggles, and self-help prospered and grew as a result.[2]

Founding Feminist Clinics

In response to agitation from doctors, lawyers, and women's groups, beginning in the mid-1960s, several states began liberalizing their abortion laws, particularly if pregnancy would impair the physical or mental health of the woman, if a child might be born with serious mental or physical defects, or if the pregnancy was the result of rape or incest. By 1972, Colorado, North Carolina, California, Georgia, Maryland, Arkansas, New Mexico, Kansas, Oregon, Delaware, South Carolina, Virginia, Florida, and Washington, D.C., allowed for abortion under such circumstances. Mississippi and Alabama also allowed for abortions in grave circumstances, though their laws were stricter. Four states, Hawaii, New York, Alaska, and Washington, passed laws allowing abortion on demand, meaning a woman did not have to demonstrate any of these special circumstances in order to terminate her pregnancy.[3]

As the restrictions on abortion began to decrease in many states in the early 1970s, self-help practitioners around the nation contemplated opening clinics to provide abortions and gynecological care for women. Some looked to existing neighborhood clinics and abortion clinics utilizing paramedics, men and women who did not hold a medical license but were trained to provide healthcare.[4] They were generally unimpressed with neighborhood clinics, because they seemed to provide the same male-dominated, paternalistic care that women encountered in mainstream medicine. One woman called the physicians at these clinics "the A.M.A. with long hair and beards."[5] Self-help practitioners tended to be much more impressed with clinics such as the one run by Dr. Frans Koome in Seattle. Koome often recruited women "off the table." That is, he asked women who came to him for procedures to join his staff as paramedics. These women performed D&Cs (a common method of abortion), did pelvic examinations and pre-abortion counseling, and stayed with patients throughout their procedures.[6]

Two Supreme Court decisions, both announced on January 22, 1973, paved the way for self-help activists around the nation to open their own clinics.[7] In *Roe v. Wade*, the court ruled that the privacy clause of the Fourteenth Amendment protected a woman's right to have an abortion. In the lesser-known companion case, *Doe v. Bolton*, the Supreme Court ruled that doctors could perform abortions outside of hospitals. This ruling, combined with *Roe*, allowed existing freestanding clinics (such as Planned Parenthood) to begin providing abortions and allowed doctors and laywomen to begin opening clinics specifically for the purpose of providing abortions.[8] Though a few self-help activists, including the West Coast Sisters, had begun providing services in clinics organized before 1973, following *Roe* and *Doe*, dozens of woman-controlled or feminist clinics sprang up around the country.[9] By 1973, there were at least thirty-five such clinics operating in the United States, on the West Coast, in the Midwest, and in the Northeast. Several more opened in the South over the next few years.[10]

Throughout the 1960s and 1970s, hundreds of feminist groups organized on the principles of egalitarianism had sprung up around the United States. Many had undertaken business ventures such as bookstores, publishing companies, record labels, restaurants, and credit unions, where they rejected traditional or "male-style" leadership and tried to make decisions by consensus. Woman-owned businesses were centers of feminist organizing, a place where women developed their politics and shared them with others. For example, women's bookstores often hosted feminist events, gave out literature on movement-related activities, and brought in speakers. Women found community in such places and cherished them as safe spaces to share their ideas and meet like-minded people.[11]

For gynecological self-help activists, feminist clinics were the logical place to carry out a feminist experiment in providing egalitarian gynecological care and abortion services. Most feminist clinics claimed to operate with a self-help philosophy. This essentially meant three things for clinic employees: they had to be committed to feminism, practice gynecological self-help themselves, and treat clients as their equals. The extent to which clinics truly enacted this philosophy varied widely across time and place.

Most of the women who opened feminist clinics immediately following *Roe* had learned about self-help at a conference or women's group and lacked formal medical training. For example, several of the women who learned about self-help from the West Coast Sisters in Los Angeles founded their own clinics in other California cities.[12] Similarly, in Greater Boston, Massachusetts, Jennifer Burgess and Cookie Avrin met at a self-help presentation in August 1973. Together with other interested women, they organized the First Annual Women's Health Conference, which brought 150 women together at the Boston YWCA. About six months later, attendees formed the Women's Community Health Center (WCHC) in Cambridge, Massachusetts and began hosting self-help groups. They then hired a doctor and began to provide abortions and birth control.[13] As other woman-controlled clinics sprang up around the country, they recruited women at local feminist events. In particular, they sought staff among the women who attended self-help presentations hosted by NOW chapters and on university campuses. In these early years, though many women saw a self-help presentation and then started clinics in their own cities, others moved across the country to join existing clinics.[14]

In most woman-controlled clinics, collective members contributed their own money to get up and running. For example, at the Emma Goldman Clinic (EGC) in Iowa City, at least one founder took out a student loan to fund the clinic, two others borrowed money from their parents, and one woman's parents paid the collective $400 to paint their house. EGC members even borrowed money from the doctor they were contracting to do abortions. He loaned them $1,000 to be paid back in one year with 6 percent interest.[15] Often, other women's groups, including established clinics and famous personalities, gave money. In 1974, the Los Angeles FWHC sent $50 per week to the new WCHC, and feminist writer and activist Robin Morgan organized a poetry reading to raise money for this clinic.[16]

Founders of feminist clinics cited their experiences of misogyny and disempowerment at the hands of physicians as motivating forces behind their decisions to establish alternative institutions. Deborah Nye traced her decision to help found EGC to the abortion she had as a seventeen-year-old. She lived in Cedar Rapids, Iowa, but the nearest doctor willing to perform the abortion was in Missouri. Though she eventually got an abortion through the help of a clergy referral network, Nye was "ticked off that [she] felt so helpless." After the abortion, Nye went to a local doctor seeking birth control pills. He informed her that unmarried women were not permitted to have them. "Doctors were controlling people's destinies," she remembered. Nye began working with a referral service called the Women's Resource and Action Center (WRAC) and started organizing self-help groups. "We could bypass legislatures and the guys and do something for ourselves. This was a way for women to take power back." When the Supreme Court legalized abortion with *Roe* in 1973, Nye and other activists convened within an hour of the decision and decided to turn WRAC into a clinic that offered abortions.[17]

Practicing Self-Help in Feminist Clinics

Gynecological self-help activists believed that women should get to know their bodies *before* they became sick or needed a doctor's care. Inside clinic walls, the self-help group became the "participatory" group where women practiced "well-woman" care. Here, women learned basic gynecological skills such as conducting cervical and breast self-exams, taking and reading a Pap smear, testing urine for pregnancy, recognizing common symptoms of sexually transmitted infections, and monitoring fertility by examining their cervixes and keeping track of their temperature.[18]

To the women who visited feminist health centers, laywomen healthworkers were the most important members of the staff.[19] Healthworkers typically had little or no medical training or experience yet occupied positions at clinics as paid staff members. Their duties included everything from taking out the trash to conducting self-exams alongside clients to assisting physicians doing abortions. New healthworkers began their training by observing more experienced healthworkers and then began assisting them in their duties. Healthworkers completed much of their training in a group setting where they could practice on each other and on themselves and share experiences.[20]

Healthworkers were supposed to model their relationship with clients on the relationship between women in self-help groups and to create an atmosphere of "sisterhood." A widely distributed self-help circular proclaimed, "If this movement is to succeed, it will—only through SISTERHOOD ... the concept of self-help stresses SISTERHOOD that makes possible the benefits from collective knowledge, collective experiences, collective training and especially the sisterly concern for one another."[21] Recognizing that a healthworker's status as an employee could still make her appear to be an authority figure, they tried to make healthworkers seem like equals to the women who came to clinics for participatory groups. Healthworkers did not wear uniforms, and they went by their first names. Feminist clinics required healthworkers to adopt a "self-help perspective" in all aspects of their work, which meant that they treated all women and all knowledge as equal. When she spoke with a woman in any context—in the clinic, on the phone, or in the community—a healthworker was supposed to share information in a nonauthoritarian manner that conveyed that the woman was the expert on her own body. Clinic literature instructed healthworkers to treat conversations with other women about healthcare as learning experiences in which they could gather anecdotal data to share with other staff and clients.[22] The idea was that the knowledge a healthworker gleaned from talking with clients and doing self-help with them was as valuable as any information she could gain from reading a medical journal or talking to a physician.[23] Most importantly, as one clinic worker at Washington Women's Self-Help explained, "When [we] . . . facilitate a self-help group, we take off our pants before we ask anyone else to."[24] Healthworkers had to be comfortable using their own bodies in order to share information about healthcare with other women. For example, most feminist clinics expected them to practice cervical self-exam on a regular basis and to demonstrate the procedure for clients. Willingness to do so was an important screening criterion for new employees. One healthworker recalled attending a meeting for women interested in working at the Tallahassee FWHC. She said that about one hundred fifty women met to see the FWHC slideshow and learn about becoming a healthworker. When the organizers reached the slide about self-exam and told the audience that conducting self-exams was part of the job, at least seventy-five women left the room immediately.[25]

No matter how much the staff emphasized an egalitarian ethos, moving gynecological self-help to a clinic setting meant compromise. First, self-help workers were paid employees. Most self-help activists subscribed to the common feminist belief that women deserved fair wages for their work, yet as wage-earning employees, they were providing a service for their clients instead of meeting them in organic, truly egalitarian, feminist "sisterhood" the way they might have done in a self-help group outside of a medical setting. Second, a clinic setting de-emphasized the political nature of gynecological self-help. Women who may not have considered themselves "political" or had an interest in women's liberation encountered self-help simply by seeking gynecological healthcare in a woman-controlled clinic. Though every woman who entered woman-controlled clinics learned about self-help, not every woman came to these clinics seeking such information. For some women, feminist health centers were simply the most convenient option for gynecological care, typically because of location. Ironically, this meant that clients were often compelled to learn about self-help whether they wanted to or not simply because they went to the nearest clinic for services.[26] Third, in order to provide medical services (especially birth control and abortions), clinic founders had to comply with the very system they sought to revolutionize: the American medical system. Federal and state laws typically required feminist clinics to hire licensed physicians to provide abortions and sometimes to write prescriptions.[27] Finding a doctor was often the most challenging part of opening a woman-controlled clinic. Even after *Roe*, many doctors, including some who considered themselves pro-choice, were unwilling to provide abortions because of the stigma attached to the procedure.[28] Many feminist clinics viewed doctors as "technicians"; they were there only to provide services that the law prohibited laywomen from providing. A doctor's status as a "technician" in a woman-controlled clinic often made it even harder for these clinics to secure their services.[29]

In spite of these necessary compromises, services provided at these health centers still stood in stark contrast to gynecological exams at doctors' offices. In a conventional gynecological appointment, a woman usually first met and interacted with her male doctor: "strip[ped] from the waist down . . . on their backs, draped, with their feet in stirrups." Celebrants of self-exam condemned the drape and stirrups and eliminated them from many clinics, arguing that they prevented women from getting visual information about their bodies and healthcare and did nothing to improve their health. One publication stated, "The drape enforces the idea that women's bodies are the domain and property of doctors." That is, lying covered up in this position prevented a woman from seeing and participating in the exam. Moreover, the drape was "an unspoken statement that we should be embarrassed and ashamed of our vaginas and reproductive organs—that they should be hidden from view."[30] Some self-help practitioners encouraged women who sought care in medical settings other than feminist clinics to discard the drape in a dramatic fashion by throwing it on the floor when the gynecologist entered the room. They suggested that if he tried to replace the drape, they should throw it on the floor again.[31] Self-help practitioners also argued that stirrups further mystified a gynecological exam and were not at all necessary for a doctor to see a cervix or feel a uterus. Forcing a woman to lie on her back with her legs awkwardly spread created an unequal power dynamic between doctor and patient and discouraged women from asking questions.[32]

In contrast, healthworkers strived to make feminist clinics comfortable and welcoming places where women felt free to ask questions and learn about their bodies. They overthrew standard terminology, protocol, and even the medical space itself. Women were not "patients"; they were clients. This further emphasized the perspective that women should visit the clinic even when they were well. The group usually began with each woman telling her medical "herstory" to the rest of the group. One FWHC publication noted that the term "herstory" emphasized the importance of "a woman's self-reporting as opposed to the 'medical history' in which the physician's secondhand impressions and so-called objective observations made with measuring devices are given much more credence." Clients had access to their own medical records during the visit and were free to verify the information in them or even to make changes. They could also make copies of their records and take them home.[33] Staff decorated with plants and soft rugs, arranged comfortable chairs in circles, and put pictures on the walls and even on the ceiling above the exam table. Women usually met in groups with other women for their visit instead of going one by one into exam rooms.[34]

Self-help revolved around sharing knowledge, so clinics often grouped clients based on the reason for their visit. For example, women who came to the clinic seeking birth control first met together as a group, as did women who needed pregnancy tests. Some groups were for lesbian women only, for menopausal women only, or for mother-daughter pairs. Other groups targeted women with a family history of cancer, women who struggled with yeast infections, or women who wanted to know more about vaginal infections. Groups discussed the prevention, treatment, and cure of common health problems using both home remedies and prescription drugs, giving attention to both self-help remedies (such as applying yogurt for a yeast infection) and medical interventions. Some learned "menstrual massage" for relieving cramps during their periods. Healthworkers demonstrated cervical and breast self-examination, and then women took turns conducting their own exams if they chose. In some participatory clinics, the group discussed birth control and did fittings for cervical caps (a nonhormonal method of barrier contraception), and even learned IUD removal.[35]

Since home pregnancy tests were not widely available yet, in many clinics, women conducted their own pregnancy tests in small groups. These groups often included women who suspected that they were pregnant and were scheduled to have an abortion later in the day or in the next few days. Other women in the same group were there to learn if they were pregnant or not and were not necessarily going to seek abortions. Feminist clinics scheduled women from both groups (those potentially seeking to terminate and those who were not) together in order to destigmatize abortion and normalize the experiences of both pregnancy and abortion. Each woman collected her own urine sample and brought it to a table. Clinic staff then gave the group instructions on placing a drop of urine on a slide, adding chemicals, and then agitating the liquid to see if it remained clear or turned cloudy. Clear indicated that a woman was not pregnant; cloudy with tiny particles meant that she was. The women in the group took turns telling each other how they felt about being pregnant; reactions ran the gamut. Testing as a group also helped some women see that they did not have to face unplanned pregnancies and abortions alone or in silence, and many found the experience both comforting and illuminating.[36] Some clinics also offered "abortion groups" just for women about to terminate their pregnancies. Typically, two healthworkers and about three to six women having an abortion that day discussed every step of the abortion procedure together.

Healthworkers encouraged group discussion, and group members provided sup-port for each other.[37]

Clinic workers understood that not every client would be comfortable with sharing her experiences with strangers, and they made some allowances for these women. Some clinics offered the option of an individual appointment with a healthworker for a woman who felt uncomfortable with or could not find time to attend a participatory clinic. This individual appointment typi-cally offered women much of the same information on self-help they could get in a participatory clinic but without the group discussion.[38] The idea was that even if a woman was not comfortable participating in a group, she could still learn about self-help techniques.[39]

When women came to the clinic for an abortion, the healthworker's job was to help them become comfortable and knowledgeable. Training manuals instructed healthworkers to describe in detail "the actual steps of the abortion and what sensations [other] women have felt." Healthworkers also explained the risks of abortion and the importance of aftercare.[40] There, the group set-ting ended, but the healthworker stayed with each client during her abortion, and her role was much like the role of the women assisting in a menstrual extrac-tion in a self-help group. In a typical menstrual extraction, at least one woman worked the entire time to ensure comfort. She offered pillows, adjusted the lighting and music, and asked questions about cramping and discomfort. Sim-ilarly, during an abortion in a clinic, healthworkers did their best to help women relax. They might offer to hold a woman's hand or massage her abdomen and remind her to breathe.[41] One training manual instructed healthworkers to "use every minute available to establish a relationship of support and trust with the woman and to help her feel in control."[42] In the event of unusual circumstances (e.g., if a woman had complications the day after an abortion and called or returned to the clinic for help on a day when no doctor was present), a health-worker also acted as a client's advocate. If necessary, she would accompany the woman to another medical facility, where she would "explain . . . procedures, solicit . . . information from medical professionals, and make . . . sure that noth-ing [was] done without the woman's complete knowledge."[43]

These were the ideals. Needless to say, clinic workers did not always meet these expectations. Clinics faced budget challenges that meant time was limited. Healthworkers did not always completely buy into the self-help philosophy, nor did clients. Attempts at maintaining a collective structure and conflicts over race and class led to burnout and disagreements. Conflicts over all of these issues played out in woman-controlled clinics across the country as women tried to balance their feminist ideals and self-help philosophy with the realities of keeping their doors open in the face of hostility from local competitors and state regulatory institutions.[44]

Conflicts over Self-Help Philosophy and Collective Feminism in Clinics

In most health centers, "feminist beliefs" were far more important criteria for hiring clinic staff than medical training or background. Jobs were often advertised under headlines reading "Feminists Wanted."[45] A survey of women's clinics in the late 1970s found that 84 percent required "feminist beliefs." How they determined these beliefs varied from clinic to clinic. Some specifically asked in the interview if a woman identified as a feminist. Others asked if she participated in any groups that advocated for women's interests, such as NOW. Many self-help practitioners also felt that it was their duty to engage in other feminist causes alongside their work in the clinic.[46]

Clinic founders thought of their attempts at collective decision making and their commitment to egalitarianism as an extension of their self-help and feminist philosophies. In theory, everyone's opinion and knowledge were valued in the clinic, just as they were in self-help groups. Each member of the clinic rotated jobs and responsibilities. Everyone attended frequent (typically weekly) business meetings that often lasted four or five hours.[47] Some clinics paid all staff equally, no matter what responsibilities they took on. Others based pay on the number of months a woman had worked for the clinic.[48]

Many feminist clinics operated independently, but some organized loosely in order to support each other. In 1975, several clinics, including three in California (closely affiliated with the West Coast Sisters), one in Detroit, and one in Tallahassee, founded the largest alliance of woman-controlled clinics, the Federation of Feminist Women's Health Centers, often simply called "the Federation."[49] In the early 1970s, staff of Federation clinics held a summer institute program to train anyone interested in self-help or in starting a woman-controlled clinic. Other clinics around the nation joined the Federation throughout the 1970s. The Federation philosophy was that a woman should be able to walk into any affiliated clinic and receive the same care that she could receive in any other Federation clinic. Similarly, healthworkers could work in any of the clinics interchangeably, so they frequently filled in at other clinics on a rotating basis. To facilitate this system, Federation clinics even organized supplies in the same manner and created a standardized method of communication.[50]

Like the West Coast Sisters, the Federation was prolific, and many of the original West Coast Sisters and their close associates published self-help books, pamphlets, and films together under the name Federation of Feminist Women's Health Centers. Downer was often the mouthpiece of the Federation, and she had a loud voice. Much of what is commonly known about this movement centers around this group. Yet her voice and even the Federation's collective voice were not the only ones in the fray. It is important to not allow them to stand for the entire self-help movement but also to recognize that they were power-ful figures. In fact, I believe that disagreements between this group and other smaller, lesser-known groups are part of what made self-help a movement rather than merely a committed group of gynecological evangelists. Much of the remainder of this chapter illuminates such disagreements, especially over the definition of feminism, and explores how they shaped the structure and course of self-help and spread awareness of it to other feminists, women's health activists, and medical practitioners.

In many Federation clinics, obvious leaders emerged in the 1970s.[51] These leaders were usually clinic founders or other women who were able to devote large amounts of time to clinic operations. In theory, though these clinics had leaders, they still tried to make decisions by consensus or committee as often as possible. In reality, this proved a challenge, and conflict over collectivism, self-help philosophy, and the meaning of feminism erupted almost from the very beginning. One such conflict played out in a very public arena: in the popular feminist periodical *off our backs*.

In 1974, a group of women from the Orange County FWHC (a Federation clinic) quit because they "could not agree with the politics" of the clinic, and they "got tired of being oppressed and told how great it was."[52] Sharon Johnson of the Federation wrote that women working in clinics may have to pat themselves on the back instead of expecting others to do it and noted that the stressful and busy nature of working in a clinic left no time for "positive reinforcement."[53] They felt that one leader, Eleanor Snow, was exerting too much control, speaking harshly, and treating the other staff as "shitworkers." The Walkout Five, as the feminist media dubbed them, were not the only women to leave the Orange County clinic that year. Turnover in all of the Federation clinics was quite high. The stressful atmosphere, the experimental nature of the clinics, and the low pay led many women to leave. Others were "squeezed out" when they did not conform to the standards of the clinic. Some women reported that only those women in whom the leaders saw a well-developed "feminist consciousness" did well in the clinics.[54]

Shortly after the Walkout Five left the Orange County FWHC, Downer published an article titled "What Makes the Feminist Women's Health Center 'Feminist'" in the *Monthly Extract*. She wrote that it was neither "total collectivity" nor "the absence of a hierarchy" that made the Federation clinics feminist. These clinics were feminist because they were "woman-controlled" and worked "toward achieving feminist goals." She argued that because any woman who worked at the FWHCs understood that her labor was "contributing solely to the . . . betterment of her sex . . . she can rest assured that she will never be exploited." Though she acknowledged that there was a hierarchy in the FWHCs, Downer insisted that there was "no labor-management split," and any woman who believed that there was such a split lacked "feminist consciousness." Further, she said, "Since a woman may not recognize where her true interest lies, she may not value the goals of the FWHC (to take over women's health care). She will then feel exploited, because the fruits of her labor are being used to further the cause that she does not identify as her own." Downer asserted that even though time constraints prevented every member of the clinic from participating in every decision, since the women making decisions "had the same interests" as the other women at the clinic, the whole group could be confident in the leaders' choices.[55]

In response to this inflammatory article, *off our backs* interviewed eleven former members of the Orange County FWHC, including a few of the women who had walked out in protest. Because *off our backs* contacted them for a quote, the Federation was aware that the article was forthcoming. Francie Hornstein of the Los Angeles FWHC wrote a letter to other clinics, within the Federation and beyond, telling them to expect a "yellow journalistic article."[56] *off our backs* published selections of the transcript of the interview. Next to the transcript, *off our backs* reprinted Downer's "What Makes the Feminist Women's Health Centers 'Feminist.'"[57]

The *off our backs* interviewees also leveled criticisms against the "Downer Dynasty" over their commitment to feminism, claiming that they exploited workers and cared more about making money from abortions than about the women they employed. The Walkout Five wrote:

> We feel that since we are challenging the FWHC on its feminism, we should give you a definition of what feminism is to us. Feminism, to us, is more than just confronting and changing the male-controlled institutions—it is a warm, strong, supporting feeling toward all women, it is sharing knowledge and experiences to work on an equal, collective level with all women to understand and fight sexism, racism, homosexism, ageism, classism, and capitalism. . . . Feminism is having an awareness of breaking down the male class system still within us, which continues to divide us. Feminism is non-exploitative. It is confronting and dealing with oppression, but it is not done by becoming more oppressive than that which we are confronting. Feminism is fighting together to change the conditions which are exploiting us; it is not gaining personal power and control for a few by exploiting other women. We think that the FWHC should remove the word "feminist" from its title, or begin to act as feminists.

The Walkout Five felt as if the leadership left them out of important decisions and took all of the desirable jobs, leaving the healthworkers to do the "shitwork." "We weren't allowed to do any of the 'glorious jobs' like calling the doctor or meeting the public without a 'proper training period' which never seemed to end," interviewee "Lorey" told *off our backs*. "We must stop the women who are taking on the exact qualities of the male power structure," said interviewee "Sue."[58] "How many times have we been told 'we don't recognize where our true interests lie' and someone will have to guide us?" asked "Shannon." "We've heard that from males and now from Carol Downer—and she doesn't even change the wording."[59]

At the crux of this fight were two questions: Who gets to define feminism? And for whom do they get to define it? Downer and other Federation clinic leaders believed that the grievances of the Walkout Five stemmed from their naïveté about feminism. They felt that the leaders needed to show the newer employees what feminism really meant. And for them, true feminism included doing "shitwork" for the benefit of the clinic. Meanwhile, the Walkout Five and other *off our backs* interviewees believed that the leaders' attempts at defining feminism for other women was, ironically, not feminist. In fact, it was paternalistic and—the worst transgression of all—male.

The *off our back* interviewees also reported that the "Downer Dynasty" claimed that they "owned" self-help. They recounted that another group of women who used to work for an FWHC tried to start their own women's center in Orange County and do self-help presentations for the public. One interviewee said that the Federation clinics believed self-help was their *"property."*[60] She also said, "No one near an FWHC would dare to hold a neighborhood self-help group without the FWHC present. Institutions here in Orange County are outspokenly fearful about having anyone but the FWHC do a self-help presentation for them."[61] Around the same time as the Walkout Five interviews, a Detroit self-help group reported that "when the FWHC established an office in this city earlier this year, we were told that continued use of the term 'self-help clinic' in our publicity would be considered legally improper."[62]

Federation clinic leaders were angry at the interviewees and *off our backs* and felt an urgent need to reply again. Hornstein said, "We have no respect for the women who wrote the article or the women who published it."[63] Downer, Rothman, and Snow wrote a lengthy rebuttal to the *off our backs* piece. It included a seventy-two-point appendix refuting various elements of the original article. They disputed the claim that the FWHCs had tried to establish a monopoly on self-help. The three women wrote, "FACT: Self-help belongs to all women." They described their efforts to help other women's groups start self-help clinics in both the United States and internationally. They also explained that they were always willing to do self-help presentations for local groups, and they encouraged these groups' "independence," since FWHC resources were limited. On the other hand, they wrote, "Starting a rival Self Help Clinic in our area would be similar to starting a rival Rape Crisis Line. There is so much work to be done that people should not go around starting projects that a women's group has already put energy into." These three leaders did not view other forms of self-help as an expansion of the services that women could offer to other women or as an improvement in the healthcare system. Instead, anyone else doing self-help in the vicinity was a "rival." Downer, Rothman, and Snow also believed that it was their duty to exercise quality control over self-help. They wrote, "We have the responsibility to see that principles of Self Help are upheld in self-help groups in our community."[64]

As the conflict played out in *off our backs*, many contributors to and readers of the popular women's periodical took sides. One article, signed by fifteen *off our backs* writers, stated, "The structure of the FWHC is inimical to the concept of self-help and feminism."[65] Some readers thought the *off our backs* interview was an "excellent bit of journalism" and a "courageous move" on behalf of the ex-workers and the publication.[66] Others saw it as "a contemptible piece of counter-revolutionary guilty jealous nonsense" and felt that *off our backs* would serve readers better by exposing the actions of misogynistic doctors and "women who are collaborating with the enemy rather than those fighting the patriarchal system."[67]

One outcome of this debacle was a re-examination of collective structure. Later that year, Hornstein wrote: "The women's movement has weakened itself by refusing to recognize leaders among our own people. We have adopted pseudo-equalitarian principles which have prevented many women from exercising their talents, abilities, and skills to their fullest capabilities. . . . We must change the concepts of strength and power into positive characteristics to which all women aspire."[68] This attitude mirrored that of many feminists who had explored collectivism in the 1960s and early 1970s. A number of scholars have examined the successes and failures of feminist collectives. Most conclude that though an egalitarian structure sometimes worked well for small groups of women with limited aims, as collectives grew larger and expanded their services, consensus-style decision making became an obstacle to progress. Woman-controlled clinics were no exception.[69] Judy Herman, a staff member at the Somerville Health Project in Massachusetts, wrote, "The women's movement cult of structurelessness has been no help at all. Maybe it works for small homogeneous consciousness-raising groups, but it's been terrible for us."[70] Two years after the walkout, Federation leaders wrote: "Some women are better suited to making decisions than others. We believe that in a structureless organization, a few people will, in fact, control the group, but in a hidden fashion. By recognizing leaders within the group, we provide the basis for making those leaders acceptable to others. The FWHC is an open-ended hierarchy."[71] All of this was in sharp contrast to their earlier stance that leaderlessness was the most feminist form of operating a business.[72]

Self-Help for Whom?

Historian Benita Roth argued famously that White women and women of color trod "separate roads to feminism."[73] Because they were often interested in combating racism, sexism, and other systems of oppression in tandem, women of color sometimes organized separately from White women, and the same holds true for other groups of marginalized women. However, even when they organized separately, women of color and White women, lesbian and straight women, working- and middle-class women often collaborated and shared strategies and theories, especially on single-issue campaigns such as abortion rights and domestic violence.[74] Even mainstream "white" organizations such as NOW included issues of poverty and racial justice in their agendas from the beginning, but a historical focus on spokeswomen (such as Betty Friedan and Gloria Steinem) and on national agendas has made such intersectional organizing difficult to see.

From the early days of the self-help movement, many gynecological self-help activists argued that women of all races, classes, and sexualities could benefit from a self-help group. However, these mostly White groups were not always adept at reaching a diverse array of women, particularly women of color and poor women, or even understanding what health issues mattered to them. Sexuality was a similar story, though White lesbian women tended to be more integrated into the ranks of middle-class White feminism (particularly because many were still in relationships with men when they joined the movement and came out later as feminism helped them further explore their sexualities).[75]

Some clinics were acutely aware of the demographic limitations of their organizations. For example, the WCHC acknowledged that the "collective poverty" of the group dictated which women could afford to work at the clinic. A full-time salary at the WCHC was $85 per week in 1977.[76] Most of the members were White, middle- to-upper-middle-class women who had the luxury of other sources of money. Many had part-time jobs in other places, some relied on their savings to supplement their income from WCHC, and others depended on support from spouses, partners, and parents.[77]

Some clinics that began with mostly White women worked hard to diversify both their staff and their clientele but were not always successful. For example, the Berkeley Women's Health Collective established a minimum number of staff positions that had to be filled by women of color.[78] Many clinic leaders and staff believed that the women who needed self-help the most were women who could not afford mainstream medical care. Some clinics were purposefully located in working-class neighborhoods in hopes of making it easier for local women to visit.[79] When Byllye Avery and her friends opened the Gainesville Women's Health Center, more than half of their abortion clients were Black women, though African Americans accounted for only around 20 percent of the Gainesville population.[80] On the other hand, the Gainesville clinic rarely attracted women of color for well-woman services even when they publicized their services in church bulletins and mailings to African American neighborhoods. Instead, young White women from the University of Florida flocked to the well-woman clinics. Avery recalled feeling disappointed about the demographics of the clients and unsure of how to better attract Black women to take part in self-help.[81] Similarly, a Tallahassee FWHC employee, Marion Banzhaf, recalled that her clinic attracted a wide range of women for abortion and birth control services, but those who attended participatory well-woman clinics were "all white all the time."[82] Francie Hornstein recalled that the same was true at the Los Angeles FWHC.[83] "We have to take responsibility for the ways we exclude other women," wrote this FWHC. Yet, in many cases, self-help activists struggled to agree about how exactly to accomplish this goal.[84]

In many clinics, conflicts about race and class reached deeply personal levels and led to irreparable fissures. One Gainesville clinic employee, Pam Smith, recalled an incident when staff member Deborah David, who Smith described as a "radical Black . . . empowerment person," argued with clinic leaders that the clinic should be doing more to bring self-help to the Black community (including men as well). Smith remembered that the clinic leaders did not respond satisfactorily, and David left.[85] Another disagreement led the entire Tallahassee FWHC to leave the Federation. This clinic, like many others, was widely involved in leftist political movements. In the late 1970s, several women from the Zimbabwe African National Union (ZANU), a guerrilla group fighting for Zimbabwean independence from colonial rule, visited Tallahassee and met with the members of the FWHC. Clinic staff showed the ZANU women the Del-Em and demonstrated self-exam. When they asked the ZANU women how the clinic could help them in their independence efforts, the ZANU women requested donations of money and sanitary napkins for women involved in guerrilla warfare. The Tallahassee clinic agreed, but they thought that they could increase their impact if they asked the Federation to provide additional help. Downer traveled to Tallahassee to discuss providing aid. She wanted to help but insisted that sending the Del-Em and literature on menstrual extraction should be part of any help the Federation offered to the ZANU women. Recalling this conflict, Banzhaf said she thought that it was fairly obvious that the ZANU women were not interested in receiving menstrual extraction technology and literature. It was not of practical use to them at that time: "Really, the guerrilla fighters needed sanitary napkins because there's no opportunity to set up a little self-help clinic out in the bush." Banzhaf recalled that in the meetings where the Federation and the Tallahassee FWHC quarreled over this issue, "'You're so racist,' got hurled around a lot" between the members of the (mostly White) group. The Tallahassee leaders felt that Downer and the Federation should respect the wishes of the ZANU women rather than maternalistically assuming that they knew what the guerrilla fighters really needed. Downer believed that it was more important to provide them with liberating technology. As a result of the disagreement, the Tallahassee FWHC decided to leave the Federation.[86]

At the Emma Goldman Clinic, the staff had several "heated" discussions over providing services for women at nearby University of Iowa. Some clinic staff feared that seeing too many women from the university did not leave enough time for them to accept "underprivileged" clients. Others were afraid that if they turned away university women seeking care in a self-help setting, then they would alienate them and lose important allies. Ultimately, the clinic decided to continue allowing students to come to the clinic. After a student's first visit, they would encourage her to make future appointments somewhere else and take a patient advocate from EGC with her. They hoped this would free up more time for low-income clients.[87]

Feminist clinic employees felt varying degrees of comfort over being "out" as lesbians. In Tallahassee, for example, Banzhaf recalled feeling that "the lesbian community was sort of separatist. . . . They thought [lesbian self-help activists] were abetting the enemy because we were helping all these heterosexual women who were getting abortions and stuff." She also recalled that "even though we were just about all lesbians who worked at the health center," clinic employees felt that they could not be out, fearing that "people wouldn't come to us if they knew we were lesbians, because especially when we were doing pelvic exams . . . that people's homophobia and heterosexism would keep them away."[88] On the other hand, in Los Angeles, Francie Hornstein felt comfortable and excited about being identifying as a lesbian at the health center. She thought it was important to set an example to other lesbian women as a woman who was comfortable talking about sex and doing self-help.[89] "The health centers were totally inclusive . . . and there were a *lot* of lesbians who worked at the health centers," Hornstein recalled. In Gainesville, Pam Smith recalled that when she started working at the clinic, every employee identified as straight. However, working with other women on issues of bodily autonomy led clinic workers to see sexuality as fluid. "Every one of us became a lesbian," Smith recalled jokingly. Indeed, many Gainesville Women's Health Clinic employees eventually came out, several leaving heterosexual marriages in the process.[90]

Most woman-controlled clinics claimed that their services were equally beneficial to both lesbian and straight women, but in practice, it is difficult to discern whether woman-controlled clinics successfully "included" their lesbian clients, no matter what the makeup of the staff was. For example, the Emma Goldman Clinic found that many lesbian women in Iowa City were uninterested in seeking care at EGC because of the clinic's emphasis on contraception and reproductive health. EGC staff disagreed with this assessment, arguing, "Lesbians were failing to make the connection between some of the medical issues and their own health needs as women, regardless of sexuality."[91] The clinic created posters, flyers, and pamphlets outlining the available health information for lesbian women and discussing the challenges they faced in receiving healthcare. Writing about this debate, in California, Hornstein wrote: "The early women's [health] movement dealt with abortion and contraception. It is naïve to think that those issues are irrelevant to us, as lesbians. They are vital to all of us who are feminists in light of the use of women's bodies by men for their purposes—from rape to population control."[92] Because of debates like these, over time, many lesbian women developed lesbian-health services within existing feminist health centers and created their own self-help groups. Women met to dialogue about topics such as coming out to a doctor and infection transmission between same-sex partners. Some groups even explored self-help methods of donor insemination and used these techniques to get pregnant.[93] In other clinics, lesbian women dialogued about the discrimination they faced from hospitals and insurance companies regarding spousal consent and coverage.[94]

"If you walked into our clinic, you were going to hear our spiel," Banzhaf recalled. Moving gynecological self-help to a clinic setting opened the practice up to women who may not have been exposed to self-help otherwise. The movement expanded rapidly as clients and healthworkers used self-help to take charge of their own healthcare. By holding participatory clinics and offering self-help-based abortion services, clinic staff dramatically extended the reach of the flourishing self-help movement. At the same time, they disseminated information about self-help and their views of feminism to every woman who walked in the door, including clients and new staff. Some women pushed back, bringing to the table a dialogue about what constituted both self-help and feminism. Self-help activists of all stripes encouraged White, middle-class, and straight activists to examine issues important to a wide array of women, and sometimes they listened. Though sometimes tensions ran high and divisions ensued, as the remainder of the book explores, many meaningful projects occurred as a result of these conversations. Consequently, the self-help movement expanded well beyond what the original participants envisioned.

3

Reforming Women's Healthcare

Self-Help as Feminist Activism

> What good is it to know how to
> recognize disease if we have a health
> system that remains unresponsive to
> prevention or to the need to provide
> adequate care for everyone?
> —Ellen Frankfort

Some feminists believed that self-help in its grandest sense meant making changes to the entire system of women's healthcare provision.[1] This meant that self-help activists often made it their business to know how other health institutions provided care for women, especially surrounding abortions and childbirth. They tried to create change by publicizing the problems with these health providers, disseminating literature speaking out against unsafe practices, and using grassroots protest tactics such as "raiding" and "inspecting" medical facilities. Others worked alongside and within mainstream medical institutions to help them provide care consistent with feminist tenets. To that end, some self-help practitioners offered the use of their own bodies in order to help train medical students in humane pelvic exams, a branch of activism that succeeded in compelling many mainstream medical institutions to offer more compassionate gynecological care.

Scholars and activists typically consider self-help separately from "infiltration" strategies such as protests and teaching medical students. I myself have long struggled with whether or not to categorize this activism as part of the self-help movement or, instead, as separate strategies used by women's health activists. I have concluded, however, that attempts to make changes to the wider system of healthcare were vital components of the self-help movement. Self-help went beyond demystifying health; it also included policing healthcare. "The information uncovered by the self-help clinic . . . could only further highlight the contradictions between the technological possibilities of providing for people's health needs now and the unwillingness of the present male supremacist state to do so," activist Collette Price wrote. "Can't we encourage the self-help clinic without giving up our struggle against the hospitals, the doctors, and the male supremacist powers that are holding us back? Or does that boggle the mind—that because we are in favor of self-help, we're also in favor of getting the power for more medical help?"[2] Feminist activists themselves referred to these "infiltration" strategies as self-help, which I believe they did strategically. "Infiltration" efforts warrant inclusion and contribute to a deeper understanding of the breadth of self-help strategies used within the movement. Additionally, they further illuminate heretofore unexplored divisions within the pro-choice movement. Though scholars have begun to examine the divisions between White women and women of color in reproductive rights movements, few have considered the divisions between "mainstream" providers of feminist gynecological care and abortion services and more radical groups such as self-help practitioners and leaders of feminist clinics.[3] Self-help activists clashed with pro-choice physicians providing care in hospitals and even in their own clinics. They were also frequently at odds with Planned Parenthood, an organization that the public had long seen as a bastion of women's reproductive rights. They even sparred with those they had once considered allies in the fight to demedicalize women's healthcare, particularly when those former allies did not meet their standards of feminist care.

Feminist Vigilantes

In 1974, five women from several of the California Feminist Women's Health Centers (FWHCs) (including Downer and Rothman) broke into the Women's Community Service Center (WCSC), an abortion clinic in Los Angeles where Harvey Karman worked, and "confiscated" various items, including exam tables and medical files.[4] According to *off our backs*, the five women believed that the medical care women received at WCSC was "substandard: the labwork inadequate, the facilities dirty, the training of paramedics poor," and that Karman was "performing experimental abortions there."[5] Local papers called the five women "a band of feminist vigilantes" who "looted an abortion clinic." The women dumped the confiscated items in the offices of the Department of Consumer Affairs and "demand[ed] . . . official action against the dangerous and illegal abortion practices occurring" at WCSC. Reportedly, they told the head of this department, "We have done what you should have done. . . . Shut him down!"[6] The city attorney of Los Angeles filed charges against the women for "trespassing and malicious mischief." In response to these charges, the FWHC said, "We did everything we did to protect the health of women."[7]

These "feminist vigilantes" sought to draw media attention to Karman's actions; they saw this as a service to women. Several FWHC employees gave interviews to the *Los Angeles Times*. "We can't wait around, risking one more woman's life," Francie Hornstein told a reporter. They also disseminated information about the raid to other feminist groups. Women from other clinics outside of California, including the Women's Community Health Center in Cambridge, Massachusetts, wrote letters supporting them, claiming that the FWHC workers showed "great courage in taking a direct, public action to draw attention to unsafe medical practices" and arguing that "women in the United States and the *world* cannot feel safe if people are allowed to practice medicine unsafely and illegally."[8]

Yet some in the women's health community did not buy the self-help activists' claims that they were acting to protect women. Merle Goldberg, a women's health activist and close associate of Karman's told *off our backs* reporters that the incident was a "vigilante tactic of Carol Downer and her brownshirt terrorists." Goldberg claimed that the self-help activists' motivations were financial. The WCSC charged significantly less for an abortion than the closest woman-controlled clinic (the Los Angeles FWHC): $40 at WCSC versus $160 at the FWHC. "Karman is just a . . . red herring," she claimed.[9]

Partly because of its association with Karman, Planned Parenthood was also a target of self-help protests. Since Margaret Sanger founded Planned Parenthood in 1921, the organization has been the leading voice in the push for access to birth control for U.S. women across classes.[10] Beginning in the 1970s, Planned Parenthood also opened clinics that provided abortions, and the organization is now the single largest abortion provider in the United States.[11] Though the organization might have seemed like a natural ally for the self-help movement, many self-help activists did not believe Planned Parenthood had a real interest in women's empowerment. Marion Banzhaf of the Tallahassee FWHC quipped, "Planned Parenthood was 'the enemy,' don't you know!"[12] While many in the pro-choice community applauded Karman's and Planned Parenthood's efforts to make abortion widely available, some self-help activists, especially Federation of FWHC members, believed that Karman's and Planned Parenthood's abortion methods were both unsafe and disempowering for women. The "Philadelphia Story" debacle had completely eroded the already fragile relationship between Karman and the Federation. While Planned

Parenthood viewed itself as a feminist organization, many self-help activists argued that because it was not woman-controlled and did not operate according to self-help principles, the organization was *not* feminist. Cataloguing the differences between feminist clinics and Planned Parenthood, reporter Jill Benderly wrote that feminist clinics had a "bigger mission: seizing our bodies" and "involving women in their own health care," while Planned Parenthood clinics "sometimes run in assembly-line fashion."[13] Banzhaf also said many self-help activists believed that Planned Parenthood clinics "weren't trying to do anything innovative or give [women] control."[14] That is, Planned Parenthood did not use lay healthworkers, nor did they encourage self-help practices such as group discussion or self-exam. "We just wrote them off as just part of the medical establishment. . . . You [would] get the same experience at Planned Parenthood that you get at the doctor's office, basically," Banzhaf recalled.[15]

Beyond just exposing the activities of Karman, self-help activists wanted to share their disdain for Planned Parenthood in general. Around the same time as the WCSC raid, self-help activists began attending Association of Planned Parenthood Physicians (APPP) conferences to "monitor" them. Though the APPP would not let them present papers at the conferences, they said that self-help activists could attend and set up a booth to disseminate information. However, in April 1974, when self-help activists Debra Law and Shelley Farber attended a conference in Memphis and set up a booth, they "were physically thrown out when they began to distribute self-help literature."[16] They reported that a guard "ransacked our booth, dragged Debra Law down the stairway of the Memphis hotel, threw her out into the street, and threw our bags and literature after her."[17]

In 1975, the Los Angeles FWHC published a list of demands "to insure that Planned Parenthood" would "function in the best interest of women." Their first objection was with the male-dominated Planned Parenthood clinic boards. "There should be the same percentage of women on the boards . . . as are in the patient loads of these clinics," they argued. The FWHC also felt that a representative of a "feminist organization" should sit on each board. Further, clinic leaders accused Planned Parenthood of not being completely open with its clients about the potentially risky nature of the contraceptives they offered.[18] They wanted Planned Parenthood to offer more literature and education on their contraceptives, particularly the "experimental nature" of some methods of birth control and the possible side effects.[19]

The rivalry between Planned Parenthood and smaller, locally based feminist clinics continued into the 1980s. In 1989, a group of representatives from women-controlled clinics across the country convened to discuss the future of their organizations. A central theme in their conversation was a concern that Planned Parenthood's growing operation was edging them out. Many faulted

Planned Parenthood for moving in just down the street from their clinics instead of opening clinics in other underserved areas nearby. The leaders of the Atlanta FWHC told the group that they were completely broke and that Planned Parenthood had plans to open a clinic in nearby Redding. "That could push us over the brink," one leader said. Francine Thompson of the Emma Goldman Clinic in Iowa City (EGC) claimed, "We are under siege by Planned Parenthood!"[20] In Iowa, there were five clinics that provided abortions at this time. Three were in Iowa City, and another was just twenty miles away from the city. Planned Parenthood wanted to open another clinic in Iowa City.[21] Responding to the EGC's concerns, the president of Planned Parenthood of Mid-Iowa, Jill June, told the press, "I think they are threatened by us and they don't need to be. . . . We don't want to compete with them." Gayle Sands of EGC told the press, "Instead of going into underserved areas, Planned Parenthood targets markets that have been set up for them by the blood, sweat, and tears of feminist clinics." Shauna Heckert of the Chico FWHC told the press, "They want to go where existing providers have already made abortion acceptable." *Women and Health* reported that Planned Parenthood told EGC that "they must either become a Planned Parenthood clinic or Planned Parenthood would set up its own abortion facility in Iowa City with a lower fee scale that would put Emma Goldman out of business." In Chico, California, Planned Parenthood's presence decreased state funding for family planning for the local FWHC.[22] Some woman-controlled clinic leaders found themselves training doctors who then left to work for Planned Parenthood and other competing clinics. "We've had to create a hostile community to Planned Parenthood by educating our clientele about what they'd lose if we weren't here. [We say] 'We're your local clinic, not a franchise.'"[23]

In a few cases when feminist clinics and Planned Parenthood tried to cooperate to stand up to grassroots anti-abortion groups, dissension still abounded. Together, they sometimes organized pro-choice events and clinic escort services, where volunteers offered moral support to women as they walked past antiabortion protesters outside of clinics. The feminist clinics often felt that they took more risks in this "activism, visibility, and community organizing," while Planned Parenthood "reaped the benefits with comparatively little energy" or "fiscal expenditure."[24]

Far from being a cohesive movement, the pro-choice community was divided over both theory and strategy. By confronting Karman and Planned Parenthood, self-help activists tried to influence the kind of care women had when they sought abortions. They saw this as part of the mission of the self-help movement. "Self-help is questioning others' decisions about what is normal for us. . . . It is fighting back. . . . It is confronting those in power," wrote the WCHC.[25] Karman and Planned Parenthood leaders believed that they too were doing work that would empower women. These self-help activists disagreed and argued that Karman and Planned Parenthood were, in fact, taking power away from women.

Self-Help Activists Bring Suit

During the 1970s, doctors around the nation expressed concerns that their profession was "under siege." In addition to competition and challenges from the women's health movement, mainstream physicians faced competition from the natural and holistic health movements. These movements, which emerged largely from counterculture groups, encouraged healthcare consumers to explore alternative healthcare providers such as chiropractors, naturopaths, and psychics, and alternative remedies such as herbs, massage, and vitamins.[26] In an address to the American College of Obstetricians and Gynecologists in 1979, President Martin Stone, MD, exhorted his colleagues to "take [the] offensive against the faddists who would supplant proven excellence within the medical profession with popular mediocrity."[27]

Because the law required feminist clinics to hire a licensed physician to perform abortions, another challenge the FWHCs faced was finding sympathetic male doctors. Feminist clinics tried to hire female doctors whenever possible, but so few women were licensed physicians that this often proved impossible. Even when they widened their net to include male candidates, many feminist clinics struggled to find doctors willing to work in a woman-controlled facility that emphasized self-help above medical intervention by a doctor. The stigma surrounding abortion made many doctors fear ridicule from their colleagues and communities and danger from extremist anti-abortion activists. Equally problematic, self-help activists had criticized physicians since the 1960s, and this disdain often led doctors to shy away from working in woman-controlled clinics. Feminist clinics sometimes prohibited doctors from wearing white lab coats and asked them to go by their first names in the clinic in order to put them on an equal plane with other employees and clients.[28] A few doctors reported that the clinics discouraged them from talking to patients at all.[29] Dr. Ben Major, who performed abortions for the Oakland clinic, reported that he stopped working there because "they wanted a person to come in and do the abortions with his mouth shut." He told a reporter that the clinic would have been better off with "a deaf-mute ob/gyn or . . . a chimpanzee to do abortions."[30]

The conflict between Emma Goldman Clinic staff and Dr. Peter North illustrates the kind of divergences that existed between healthworkers and doctors in many feminist clinics. When the clinic opened in 1974, EGC contracted North to provide abortions. EGC Collective members were nervous about his attitude even before the clinic opened its doors. First, North told the staff that he did not want them present during the actual abortion procedures. Collective members also reported that he was generally "unresponsive" and "vague about time and energy commitment." One Collective member noted that the clinic was "unfortunately dependent on North for time allowances, which, when dealing with an apparently lazy male, is disgustingly restrictive and oppressive."[31] Even after North had worked at EGC for a couple of years, the power struggle continued. For example, in 1976, Collective members reported that North often criticized other staff in front of clients and spoke to clients in a way that Collective members found offensive.[32] One Collective member, Susan Miller said that a client was "brought to tears" by North's attitude during a difficult pelvic exam.[33] She recounted that North raised his voice and angrily told the client that her "muscles were so tight he couldn't do a pelvic." Miller noted that this was not the first time North had behaved this way and maintained that he was reacting in response to "his own frustration at being 'resisted' by the woman's body" and his feeling that he should be in a position of authority over the client.[34] Another healthworker reported that North was often "hostile, punitive, impolite, patronizing, impossible to deal with . . . acting like a classic male pig doctor." She was tempted to leave the clinic because of his behavior.[35] The clinic advertised for another doctor in both feminist and medical periodicals, but only a handful of doctors responded. Those who did respond proved equally incompatible, usually because they seemed patronizing. After many months struggling to find a doctor and dealing with North, the clinic even considered setting up a scholarship to help a woman medical student in exchange for her agreeing to work in the clinic after she graduated. In spite of these differences, EGC continued to employ North, because they could not find anyone else more suitable. Their frustration with his attitude continued, and the women continued framing his behavior as typically "male."[36]

Feminist clinics butted heads with physicians who did not work for them too; one such struggle came to a head in Tallahassee, Florida, in events that made national headlines. The Tallahassee FWHC employed two doctors who were also associated with Tallahassee Memorial Hospital. The FWHC offered first-trimester abortions for $150, while most other local doctors charged between $200 and $250. About a year after the FWHC opened, the *Tallahassee Democrat* compared the fees of an FWHC abortion with the fees of local doctors, noting the large discrepancy. Citing an interview with FWHC director Linda Curtis, the article also favorably described the clinic's feminist self-help philosophy, emphasizing that "women set the pace for what goes on." Local doctors felt that the article was in poor taste because it advertised abortion services, an uncommon practice at the time. Several Tallahassee doctors began to hassle the two doctors who worked at the FWHC, and within a month both of them quit. The ob-gyn staff at Tallahassee Memorial Hospital put out a statement saying that the physicians the hospital employed "should not be associated with agencies that advertise their medical services." They informed the FWHC that they were opposed to their practice of holding self-help clinics and to their political activism around the issue of abortion. In order to continue providing services, the Tallahassee FWHC hired doctors from out of town. Subsequently, the executive director of the Florida Board of Medical Examiners advised at least one of the out-of-town doctors to discontinue his work with the FWHC. He warned that any doctor associating with the FWHC was putting his career in danger if he continued to work there.[37]

"Vigilante" tactics such as raiding Karman's clinic were only one element of self-help political activism; playing by "the man's" rules and working within the existing system by taking their complaints to the courts was also a valued strategy. In October 1975, the Tallahassee FWHC filed suit against a group of local doctors, claiming that they were hindering the FWHC's ability to provide healthcare.[38] Lolly and Jeanne Hirsch wrote in the *Monthly Extract*, "When the medical establishment woke up and recognized the women were successfully providing good care for women, the monopolists went into action to rid themselves of competition."[39] In *Feminist Women's Health Center, Inc. v. Mahmood Mohammad, M.D., et al.*, the FWHC charged that the doctors were violating the Sherman Anti-trust Act (which prohibits monopolies and other anticompetitive practices) by conspiring to boycott the FWHC, fixing prices for abortions, and monopolizing the abortion provision market in Tallahassee.[40] The Tallahassee FWHC and their supporters around the nation saw their court fight as a continuation of the fight self-help activists had been waging outside of court since before *Roe v. Wade*.[41] To them, this was just one more incident in a long history of doctors trying to control women's healthcare.[42] Hirsch and Hirsch also wrote, "Tallahassee's health system is a microcosm of the pervasive system of control that the American Medical Association now has on this country's health system."[43] Throughout the suit, the FWHC suspected foul play from the court. In October 1976, the judge dismissed the case merely hours before jury selection was scheduled to begin. Codirector of the clinic Linda Curtis told a reporter that she suspected that the American Medical Association was behind the judge's decision to throw the case out. Women picketed at the federal courthouse carrying signs that read, "Who owns the Judge?"[44]

The FWHC appealed their case to the Fifth Circuit Court, which ruled that federal courts had jurisdiction and that a jury should try the case. The FWHC considered this ruling a triumph in itself, because the court "den[ied] the doctors' claim that they should be subject only to professional peer regulation." As a result of this ruling, the physicians offered to settle out of court in order to avoid further negative publicity. The FWHC accepted a settlement of $75,000 because they "recognize[d] that they [could] not expect to receive justice from the legal system." The doctors involved pledged to provide services for the FWHC and agreed to allow the clinic to easily transfer women to the hospital in case of emergency.[45] Like the "Great Yogurt Conspiracy," *Feminist Women's*

Health Center, Inc. v. Mahmood Mohammad, M.D., et al. was a victory in the fight for the right to practice self-help in a clinic setting. And once again, as news of the case spread, support came from many corners of the feminist movement.

Moreover, this case was part of a broader effort to rein in physician control over healthcare. Shortly after the FWHC filed suit, in December 1975, the Federal Trade Commission (FTC) determined that the American Medical Association as a whole was "prevent[ing] doctors and medical organizations from disseminating information on the prices and services they offer, severely inhibiting competition among health care providers." That is, they were keeping consumers from learning truthful information about prices and insurance coverage and thus restricting trade. This issue went all the way to the Supreme Court, and the FTC prevailed. This was huge; before this time, the "learned professions," including physicians, had been exempt from antitrust laws; self-help activists were a part of overturning this practice.[46]

Tallahassee Memorial Hospital Inspection

Some self-help activists also sought to influence the care women received when they gave birth. In 1977, a group of women's health activists from across the United States convened at the Southern Women's Health Conference in Gainesville and formed Women Acting Together to Combat Harassment (WATCH), a group devoted to investigating women's health facilities.[47] The following year, more activists from woman-controlled clinics in Vermont, New Hampshire, Florida, Michigan, Georgia, and California, as well as several representatives of the feminist media, joined WATCH in Tallahassee for a series of workshops. They dialogued about the hostility of mainstream medicine toward feminist clinics and about the kind of care that women received in mainstream facilities.[48]

Several members of WATCH decided to perform an "inspection" of the maternity ward of Tallahassee Memorial Hospital. Many local WATCH members had been at odds with the hospital for years as a result of the antitrust suit. Reports on what occurred during the inspection vary. Supporters called it a "peaceful consumer inspection," while opponents depicted it as an "invasion."[49] According to WATCH, the inspection uncovered a number of unsatisfactory practices in the hospital, which they planned to make public. The thirty inspectors, including a filmmaker and her cameraman, walked in the front door of the hospital and went directly to the fourth floor to see the delivery and postpartum wards and the nursery.[50] First, they saw babies, separated from their mothers, crying in a soundproof nursery. According to hospital policy, the new mothers could have chosen "rooming in," keeping the newborn's crib next to the mother's bed. However, the nurses on duty informed the inspectors that most mothers were in too much of a postdelivery, drug-induced haze to request this option. The inspectors also reported that they found containers of a cleaning chemical known to cause brain damage in newborn babies on the obstetrical ward. They described the postpartum area of the hospital as "prison-like," because mothers' movements were limited to this area. Finally, they reported the use of internal electronic fetal monitors. Members of the feminist community, along with others interested in childbirth reform, had been protesting the use of such fetal monitors for some time, arguing that they "fostered [an] emergency mentality" and led doctors to overuse cesareans.[51] The WATCH report described the internal monitor as "a small electrode . . . screwed into the skull of the baby while it is still in the mother's uterus."[52] No one openly objected to their visit until the WATCH members entered the nursery. At that point, they were asked to leave, which they did.[53] Tallahassee police subsequently arrested four of the WATCH inspectors: Carol Downer, Ginny Cassidy-Brinn, Janice Cohen, and Linda Curtis.[54]

The arrests and ensuing trials attracted a great deal of national publicity and inspired many feminists and health professionals to comment and act. When she heard of the arrests, Simone de Beauvoir wrote: "This reminds me of very old stories. For centuries, women knew how to cure diseases and help pregnant women . . . but men had POWER. So they said those women were witches and burned thousands and thousands of them. Are we still in the Middle Ages?"[55] In response to the arrests, women's health activists around the nation planned other hospital inspections and investigations of childbirth practices in mainstream medical establishments. Some members of the medical community also supported the activists. Dr. Louis Gluck, director of neonatal and perinatal medicine at the University of California, San Diego Medical Center, wrote a letter to the prosecutor urging him to drop the charges, stating that the prosecution's claim that the women had endangered the lives of the infants by entering the nursery was simply incorrect. Had the activists tried to pick up the babies with contaminated hands, then they would have placed the babies in danger, rationalized Gluck. He went on, "I have strong feelings about the haphazard way that technology is being used in hospitals across the country, and so I support these women's right to inspect hospitals and demand changes." Women from around the country came to support the WATCH women during the three-day trial.[56]

Many feminists believed that the trial was unfair from the very beginning. The presiding judge, Charles D. McClure, would not allow the defense to present any testimony on whether entering the nursery without scrubbing and gowning was harmful to infants. Deeming that this evidence was not relevant to the charge of criminal trespass, McClure also refused to allow evidence demonstrating that the presence of groups visiting the hospital after visiting hours was a common occurrence at Tallahassee Memorial. A WATCH newsletter reported, "It is obvious that this prosecution was undertaken to punish those associated with the Tallahassee FWHC because of their strong differences with the local medical association and, indeed, with Tallahassee Memorial itself." The defendants and their supporters saw the actions of Tallahassee Memorial as retaliation for the antitrust suit. Because the incident occurred after hours, the four women were found guilty of trespassing.[57] Two women received fines of $500 and thirty days in jail; the other two received $1,000 fines and sixty-day jail sentences.[58] Yet again, however, their actions had brought national attention to the self-help movement.

Pelvic Teaching Program

While some groups used combative tactics to confront those in power, other self-help activists took a more collegial approach. Historically, medical students had learned to conduct pelvic examinations on plastic models and anesthetized women. Often, no one asked anesthetized women for their consent. Beginning around 1972, Dr. Robert Kretzschmar in the Department of Obstetrics and Gynecology at the University of Iowa hired several women who were working toward advanced degrees at the university to serve as "pelvic models." These women underwent pelvic exams and gave feedback to students. Other medical schools also quickly began experimenting with this model.[59]

In 1975, healthworkers at Women's Community Health Center (WCHC) agreed to participate as models for Harvard Medical School as part of the Pelvic Teaching Program or PTP. The program was a source of controversy at the WCHC from the very beginning. Some staff members argued that it would simply reinscribe the existing power dichotomy between women and doctors by teaching physicians how to "manage" their women patients without actually changing the power structure. Others argued that this incremental step in changing doctor behavior was an important element of reforming the medical system from the inside. A few were also happy to see some of the money available to medical schools funneled into the women's health movement, as each model received $25 per session. Four or five medical students practiced pelvic exams on each participant during each session. In theory, the active participants, who let the students know whether or not what they were doing was uncomfortable or even painful, offered "a counterbalance to institutionalized attitudes toward women as passive recipients of medical care."[60]

Harvard Medical was very pleased with the arrangement, but after a few sessions, the PTP participants decided that they were not satisfied. The PTP models felt that their feedback on the exams was barely considered; students were more interested in the feedback from the observing professor. The PTP models reported that when they made comments other than "you're hurting me," students saw them as "distracting or trivial."[61] The group began to feel that though they were "ensuring more humane and better exams for women, they were also solidifying physicians' power over women by participating in training sessions." Rather than altering the current medical system, they feared they were accommodating and strengthening it, so they changed tactics.[62] Hoping to get even more women's perspectives, the WCHC expanded the program to include women who did not work at the clinic, for a total of eleven models. The requirement for participants was prior participation in a self-help group and commitment to the WCHC philosophy of self-help. Under this new protocol, two "feminist instructors" from WCHC (instead of a licensed doctor) taught groups of four or five medical students. At least one student in each group had to be a woman. Any licensed physicians present had to observe silently. The instructors even demonstrated self-exam for the medical students. They created a pamphlet titled "How to Do a Pelvic Examination," and Harvard Medical agreed to use it.[63]

As part of the new protocol, the eleven PTP women began meeting separately to do self-help sessions together. The group shared information with each other on how to do a comfortable pelvic exam.[64] They also discussed criticisms of the program, talked about any negative encounters that occurred during the teaching sessions, and shared their feelings about serving as models. Some women reported that the medical students made uncomfortable jokes or behaved as if they thought the lesson was unimportant. At this point, the PTP and the WCHC began dialoguing more about "reform versus radical change." They agreed that, as implemented thus far, the PTP was not creating radical change in the medical institution.[65]

The PTP wanted to change the program again, this time more dramatically, in order to emphasize their self-help philosophy. First, they asked Harvard Medical to limit the program to women medical students. They felt that as part of the self-help movement, the PTP must focus on reciprocal sharing between women. They also hoped that this move would force the medical community to consider whether men should be providing gynecological care for women at all. The members of the PTP felt that the occasional embarrassment and exploitation that they had felt because of the male students would no longer be a problem under this new system. Next, they also asked to expand the teaching groups beyond medical students so that other hospital personnel and consumers could participate as well. PTP members felt that this move would address the "hierarchy and elitism among medical care providers and between providers and consumers." Third, the PTP requested that the "instructors" in the group should sometimes act as models and vice versa, thereby breaking down the hierarchy within the group. Fourth, the group wanted to expand their sessions from one to four to allow time for the group to discuss the politics of medical care and to perform self-exam. Finally, the group raised their fees significantly. They asked for $750 for four sessions. In spite of the fact that other local universities, including Tufts and Boston University, had recently begun inquiring about the program, after the PTP demanded these changes, no medical schools agreed to work with them. They taught no further sessions.[66]

The PTP further highlighted the question of separation versus infiltration. Was the purpose of self-help to create separate, feminist spaces or to reform existing institutions? As one PTP participant argued, the PTP's third iteration promoted a political agenda: "to eradicate hierarchy and professionalism" in medicine. The medical establishment (or at least Harvard Medical and other local universities) was not receptive to this kind of overhaul. PTP members wrote that they feared programs like this one were "contributing to the support of a health care system that needs *radical* change." Because of this fear, they "*strongly* discourage[d] other groups of women from participating in similar programs." After this experience, PTP members and WCHC staff wondered if it was even possible to make changes to the mainstream medical establishment.[67] What, then, self-help activists wondered, was the answer? Should they turn exclusively to their own institutions? Retreat to self-help groups and try to avoid established medicine altogether?

"What good is it to know how to recognize disease if we have a health system that remains unresponsive to prevention or to the need to provide adequate care for everyone?" wrote feminist journalist Ellen Frankfort in 1972. This was a question many self-help activists wrestled with. Further, they wondered what to do about the existing system. Using a variety of tactics, including protests, court cases, inspections, raids, media attention, and cooperation with medical officials, some worked to alter this system. They considered this an extension of their role as self-help activists, a way to help a wider array of women. Long frustrated with institutional medicine, though, as the next chapter explores, some feminists worked to create completely separate structures and to avoid institutional medicine whenever possible.

4

Radicalizing Healthcare

Advanced Uses for Gynecological Self-Help

> All one needs is her own speculum and
> this book (and . . . a self-help clinic). . . to
> take care of most problems that arise.
> —*off our backs* contributor, Fran Moira

Some self-help activists believed that the purpose of self-help was to create separate groups to empower women to take care of their own health. These activists believed that it was impossible to create change within mainstream
medicine, so they chose to act outside of it whenever possible. In contrast to
the "liberal" approach of changing institutions from within, we might view
these tactics as more "radical."

This activism took place in the context of many other leftist experiments in
acting "separately." Most famously, groups like the Washington, D.C.–based
lesbian separatist Furies Collective tried to organize their entire lives separate
from mainstream institutions. They lived and worked together, eschewing
patriarchal and heteronormative systems of both work and family. Feminists
established their own bookstores, credit unions, and dozens of other institutions where they promoted feminist ideology while simultaneously offering
jobs and services to women. Separatism was also in keeping with Black Power

activism, which encouraged the creation of businesses and institutions that furthered Black values and valued racial pride.[1]

Efforts to create separate self-help institutions went well beyond forming clinics. Some feminists created "advanced" self-help groups where they experimented with "fertility consciousness" (observing changes in their cervical mucus in order to control the timing of their pregnancies), fit cervical caps, and performed donor insemination in their homes. Groups of older women investigated and informed others about aging and menopause. These groups revealed that it was possible for women to control their own reproduction without assistance from medical providers, but there were limits to how much care they could provide in this fashion.

Cervical Caps

Beginning in the late 1970s, a number of woman-controlled clinics and mainstream physicians began offering the cervical cap, a method of barrier birth control similar to a diaphragm.[2] Whereas a diaphragm is wide and flat and stays in place because of the tension in its spring rim, a cervical cap is thimble-shaped and fits tightly over the cervix, where it creates suction so that it will stay in place.[3] As with the diaphragm, versions of the cervical cap originated centuries ago. Historical records from ancient Sumatra described caps made of molded opium and cast aluminum.[4] Italian author and renowned "womanizer" Giacomo Casanova reported giving his lover half of a squeezed lemon to use as a cervical cap in the mid-eighteenth century. As birth control activists such as Margaret Sanger and Emma Goldman promoted barrier methods of contraception in the early twentieth century, the modern, flexible version of the cap became popular in the United States and Europe.[5]

As women became increasingly aware of complications with oral contraceptives (the Pill) and intrauterine devices (IUDs) in the 1970s, they looked for alternative methods of birth control. When the Pill was introduced in the United States in 1960 in a high-dose formula, it seemed like a miracle drug to many women. However, women soon began reporting serious side effects, including blood clots and strokes. Outrage grew among members of the women's health community as they realized how uninformed most women who took the Pill were about the potential side effects. In response to the uproar about the Pill, many 1970s physicians began promoting IUDs, particularly the recently developed Dalkon Shield, claiming that they were a safer alternative. Young women and women of color were especially encouraged to try the Dalkon Shield because many providers believed they were unreliable pill takers. It quickly became clear that the Dalkon Shield held dangers of its own. Women began developing serious infections; at least seventeen women died, and around two hundred thousand reported physical injuries, miscarriages, and sterilizations.

Self-help activists became interested in the cap as a result of women's contin-ued dissatisfaction with other birth control methods.[6] As with other methods of barrier contraception, a woman could decide for herself when and how to use the cervical cap. The side effects of the device were minimal, because, unlike hormonal birth control (such as the Pill), it did not interact with a woman's body chemistry in any way. Unlike an IUD, a woman could decide when to insert and remove the cap completely on her own.[7] Many women preferred the cap over the diaphragm because they could leave it in longer (up to three days at a time) and because, unlike a diaphragm, once a cap was inserted, the wearer and her sexual partner typically did not notice its presence.[8] Healthcare pro-viders around the country, particularly healthworkers in woman-controlled health centers, began seeking more information about the cap. They ordered caps in bulk from Europe as well and began fitting their clients with them. The New Hampshire Feminist Health Center reported that by 1980, there were about two-hundred cap fitters in the United States and that between ten thou-sand and fifteen thousand women had tried the cap.[9]

Around this time, the Food and Drug Administration (FDA) decided that the cap needed to undergo a series of clinical trials to determine its safety and effectiveness as a birth control device. They pulled the cap from the market in 1980 but allowed several U.S. cap fitters, including lay healthworkers in woman-controlled clinics and members of independent self-help groups, to continue fitting caps and report their findings to the FDA. This was the first time in his-tory that the FDA had allowed layperson access to a form of unapproved con-traception outside of its own clinical trials.[10]

In 1981, a group of feminist clinics and self-help groups undertook a series of studies of the cap's safety and effectiveness.[11] Many such groups had mem-bers who had been using or providing the caps for several years before FDA clas-sification. They believed it was a safe alternative to the Pill or IUDs. As health activist and author Barbara Seaman told the *New York Times*, many women's health activists thought it was "senseless for the FDA to put restrictions on the cap, which is such a benign device, while the Pill and IUD are unrestricted." In order to substantiate this claim and try to keep the cap on the market, some groups continued their studies for as many as four years. They gathered and reported extensive data from the clients they provided the cap for. Though many self-help activists had long seen their activities as a contribution to feminist research, this was the first time that self-help practitioners as a group contrib-uted significantly to a large-scale federal research effort.[12]

To collect data, each participating clinic and self-help group held self-help sessions in which women tried on different sizes and types of caps.[13] The Los Angeles FWHC offered "cervical cap parties" for fittings. Healthworkers and other self-help activists led self-help sessions in the homes of interested women. They offered free or reduced rates on the cap for women who organized and hosted the parties.[14] Some women, including the Washington Women's Self-Help Group, moved their private self-help groups into neighborhood clinics and set up shop solely for the purpose of fitting caps. They held educational teach-ins on using the caps. Using speculums, lights, and mirrors, women fit them-selves with the proper cap with some assistance from healthworkers.[15] Some clinics, such as the Bread and Roses Women's Health Center in Milwaukee, offered individual cap fittings as an alternative to a group setting and allowed women to bring their partners to the fitting.[16] Self-help groups practiced self-exam at the fittings and at home to determine the cap's effect on their bodies. Many groups asked women to share their findings by returning to recurring meetings. For others, women were on their own after the initial fitting but reported their findings through mail-in surveys. Many had previously used a diaphragm or other form of birth control, so meetings often consisted of com-paring one form of contraception to another. One study, conducted by the Atlanta FWHC and six self-help groups located mostly in the South, surveyed 1,650 women after three months of using the cap. In that time frame, they found that the cap was 93 percent effective at preventing pregnancy for women who used it consistently and correctly. Most women noticed very few side effects at all and reported general satisfaction with it.[17]

Undertaking research on this scale and in conjunction with the FDA created new obstacles for self-help activists. Most self-help practitioners were inexperi-enced at conducting research within the confines of institutionalized American science. In order to participate and continue providing the cap, feminist clinics needed to have access to an Institutional Review Board (IRB). IRBs, which review and approve research conducted with human subjects, are typically asso-ciated with larger institutions, such as universities and hospitals. In order to get access to an IRB, feminist clinics dealt with a great deal of red tape. Untrained in the ins and outs of the system, clinics and their satellite self-help groups often found themselves unintentionally out of compliance with the law. Some self-help activists believed that this red tape was the FDA's way of punishing the women's health movement for their earlier cooperation with other women's health groups' efforts to create legislation to increase the safety of other birth control methods such as the Pill and the Dalkon Shield IUD. In spite of these hurdles, women in self-help groups and feminist clinics around the nation con-tinued fitting the cap and reporting their findings until the mid-1980s.[18]

As with the Pelvic Teaching Program, self-help activists offered their own bodies as tools for a feminist research project. The Emma Goldman Clinic (EGC) hired "models" who had experience using the cap in order to teach other women to do cap fittings. Typically, the models worked in the clinic already, but they could earn extra money by acting in this capacity: $100 for the first session and $75 for every subsequent session. The model inserted her own spec-ulum, and then training participants took turns practicing putting the cap over her cervix. Typically, each model worked with two women in training at a time. About four women acted as models at once so that trainees could have experience fitting caps for women with a variety of body types. Models worked for about two or three hours at a time. Of course, being a cap model could quickly become uncomfortable. The clinic advised the models to drink lots of water and take sitz baths immediately after a training session. Much like the women who served as PTP models, cervical cap models allowed providers to use their bodies as a kind of primer or textbook. They believed that fitting a cap on an actual woman who could provide feedback and guidance was much more effective than using a plastic replica or just learning from written instructions.[19] Though self-help activists were most interested in training other laywomen to do fittings, at least one self-help group trained doctors to fit caps. Self-help activist Rebecca Chalker and two other women rented space from a "liberal doctor" in New York and trained the entire ob-gyn cohort at Columbia Medical School.[20]

The cap never became incredibly popular in the United States, probably because it had a relatively high failure rate and was not available in many gynecologists' offices. Yet, the cervical cap studies undertaken by self-help practitioners further illuminate tensions over the self-help movement's relationship to institutionalized medicine. Self-help activists believed that the cervical cap was an empowering contraceptive device because women could control its use themselves. They recognized that a diaphragm offered many of the same benefits but wanted women who were dissatisfied with diaphragms to have the option of another barrier method. Though she needed a medical provider in order to get it, once a woman had a cervical cap, there was no need to continue interacting with a physician. Possessing a cervical cap imbued a woman with a kind of power that she did not have when she relied on a doctor to write a prescription for birth control pills every month or to insert and remove an IUD when he saw fit.

However, once the FDA began to limit the use of cervical caps, feminist clinics and self-help groups had to interact with some of the very institutions that they viewed as the enemy in order to continue providing the cap. They tried to influence the FDA from within the confines of its own study. At perhaps its most radical, feminism meant severing ties with the institutions feminists viewed as patriarchal and oppressive. Yet in this case, in order to create a radical alternative for women, self-help activists had to cooperate with the federal government.[21]

Fertility Consciousness and Donor Insemination

In the 1950s, two Australian doctors, Evelyn and John Billings, backed by the Catholic Church, developed the Ovulation Method (OM) of "natural" birth control, sometimes called the Billings Method. This method is often confused with the "rhythm method," where a woman charts her menstrual cycle, determines its average length, and avoids having sex during the most fertile days. The Billings themselves were Catholics who did not believe in chemical or barrier methods of birth control. Like many other Catholics, they were dissatisfied with the failure rate of the rhythm method and sought another method of "natural" birth control. The husband and wife couple discovered that over the course of a menstrual cycle, the mucus of the cervix undergoes observable changes. Couples observing these changes carefully could control their reproduction quite efficiently. Billings OM classes became popular in the United States in the mid-twentieth century, often encouraged by the Catholic Church.[22]

In Cambridge, Massachusetts, in the late 1970s, a group of self-help activists sought to further remove their fertility from institutional control; ironically, in order to do so, they co-opted a method of birth control promoted by the Catholic Church. In an era when contraception was becoming increasingly medicalized, instead of interacting with doctors, pharmaceutical companies, and the government, these women sought to control their reproduction the "natural" way. These activists were mostly affiliated with the WCHC and the Rising Sun Feminist Health Alliance, the largest coalition of woman-controlled clinics and self-help activists outside of the Federation of Feminist Women's Health Centers. Rising Sun was based in the northeastern United States, from Maryland to Maine, and as far east as Pennsylvania. They met semi-annually, mostly to network and offer moral and monetary support for each other's efforts.[23] In "fertility consciousness" groups, women from WCHC and Rising Sun put a feminist spin on OM.

When they learned of this method, self-help activists took issue with the political and religious context in which OM was developed and practiced. They argued that OM was intended to promote and strengthen "traditional" marriage and emphasize motherhood as woman's "natural" role. They believed that its developers and promoters did not intend it as a method of woman-controlled birth control. In fact, self-help activists argued, its promoters intended for the women who used OM to remain as ignorant as possible about the science behind the method. They cited a phrase commonly used in OM trainings, "Keep it simple, stupid," or KISS, as evidence that Billings Method promoters encouraged teachers to share as little information with their students as possible.[24] After attending a Billings Method conference, Jill Wolhandler from WCHC reported that "the political atmosphere was very Catholic—pro-nuclear family, anti-abortion, anti-sexuality." She told other members of Rising Sun that the conference was rife with tensions between the traditional Billings instructors and the feminist groups.[25]

The WCHC and Rising Sun groups believed that the Billingses and the Catholic Church wanted to keep strict control over OM. They saw the formation and trademarking of the World Organization / Ovulation Method / Billings

(WOOMB) as further evidence. One participant argued that the church was "trying to gain a monopoly over selection and training of teachers by requiring and controlling a teacher certification process. Criteria included acceptance of and adherence to the moral philosophy of WOOMB."[26]

In "fertility consciousness" self-help groups, women redirected what they saw as a moralistic message of OM supporters.[27] In particular, they tried to "recognize and value sexuality as separate from reproduction."[28] They shared information about other methods of birth control and compared notes on their side effects and effectiveness. The purpose was not to promote OM, but to explore it, in a self-help setting, as one among many possible birth control options.[29] Self-help activists argued that fertility consciousness as a method of birth control "completely frees a woman of dependence on a medical professional in matters regarding her fertility." Further, they wished to contextualize this method as part of a long history of women controlling their own fertility. Though most of the members of the group had learned about fertility consciousness because of the increasing popularity of the Billings Method, they began exploring its deeper roots. As fertility consciousness practitioner Susan Bell wrote: "The fact that cervical mucus is related to fertility was well known before modern times. Not only the Bantu people in East Africa, but also the Native American Cherokee people possessed this knowledge.... Mothers passed information about cervical mucus to their daughters. Disruption of these and other cultures by imperialism has broken down traditional communication networks and values. Countries like the United States have further encouraged the breakdown of traditional communications by exporting profitable and sometimes dangerous medical birth control devices to control population throughout the world." Understanding that knowledge of fertility consciousness had been suppressed furthered self-help activists' belief that recapturing this knowledge was a crucial element of feminist bodily empowerment.[30]

After reading a WCHC article on fertility consciousness, John Billings wrote to the WCHC expressing both his happiness that the group was exploring OM and his disagreements. He agreed that OM was "certainly not a Catholic method," emphasizing that it was backed by "expert, meticulous scientific research." Billings wrote that he fully supported use of OM as a means of women's liberation, noting that he and his wife were especially interested in seeing the method used for this purpose, because they had five daughters of their own. He emphasized that when women attended OM classes at his teaching center in Australia, they were not required to accept Catholic teachings or even have knowledge of them. Billings took issue with the WCHC's characterization of the KISS method, defending the necessity of that method as a way to encourage teachers not to overload women with unnecessary information. "We are anxious to avoid the situation where the woman goes away bewildered and disheartened rather than informed," he wrote. He also argued that it was important for OM teachers to ensure that they taught couples enough about the method to make them "autonomous and not dependent."[31]

Self-help activists also thought that fertility consciousness was a useful way for women to become more familiar with their own bodies and gain greater bodily autonomy, much like menstrual extraction. Each time the Cambridge area group met, they conducted self-cervical exams in order to observe the changes in their cervical mucus that would indicate fertility. They chose the name "fertility consciousness" in order to emphasize that "this information has a broader applicability than birth control."[32] They argued that the knowledge about her body that a woman gained by practicing fertility consciousness was "every woman's right."[33] They saw fertility consciousness as a "self-help tool" because it "allow[ed] all women greater body awareness," and some believed that even women who did not need birth control would find it "empowering."[34]

Fertility consciousness could also be useful for women trying to conceive; some lesbian self-help activists in particular found this knowledge invaluable. Francie Hornstein grew up knowing she wanted to have children, and she had no interest in being with a man. Shortly after she began participating in women's liberation activities in Iowa City in the early 1970s, she began to think about how she could have a child. At the time, she did not know any other women, even feminists, who were talking about having kids on their own or with women partners. Then Hornstein met the women from the Los Angeles FWHC and decided to move to California to work there. She said that once she learned about self-help and fertility consciousness, "the technology became obvious."[35] She realized that just as self-help activists had taught themselves to do Pap smears, fit cervical caps, check IUDs, and perform menstrual extractions, they could learn to inseminate themselves. They started by reading the available medical literature and talking with sympathetic medical professionals. Then Hornstein, her partner Ellen Peskin, and their friends dialogued in groups about their own bodies and experiences and about the information about ovulation patterns that self-help practitioners had gleaned by attempting fertility consciousness.[36]

Around this time, so-called assistive reproduction techniques were on the rise. Over the course of the twentieth century, various medical professionals had undertaken experiments to "artificially" inseminate their female patients, resulting in thousands of successful pregnancies. Many doctors and patients acted secretly; this "personal" technology was largely unregulated. In most cases, this technology was used by married couples who were struggling to get pregnant; doctors simply inserted a husband's semen into his wife's vagina or uterus in order to increase the chances that the sperm reached the egg. Some evidence suggests also that a few doctors had been secretly using donor sperm, perhaps even without the couple's consent or knowledge, in order to help a woman conceive. In the 1970s, sperm banks rose in popularity as more doctors and their patients experimented with using frozen sperm for insemination.[37]

Self-help donor insemination was largely uncharted waters when Hornstein and Peskin attempted it. They were "forging this new ground of how to do this as lesbians," Peskin recalled.[38] Though the exact origins of experimentation with "at home" donor insemination are unclear, it seems that a number of women in the United States and elsewhere began exploring it seriously in the early 1970s.[39] They drew on the knowledge of their bodies gleaned through participating in self-help groups and reading medical texts. They also used information from farmers, ranchers, and scientists who had successfully practiced artificial insemination on animals since at least the fourteenth century.[40]

Hornstein and Peskin both successfully used self-help methods to get pregnant. Hornstein went first, about four years before Peskin. Recalling the process, Hornstein said, "I always had this worry in the back of my head that there was something special you had to do, and would this really work? And was it really that easy? Just collecting the sperm and putting it in my vagina?" As it turned out, "collecting the sperm" was the difficult part. They found a friend willing to donate. Using fertility consciousness to get the timing right, they waited until Hornstein was most fertile. The first time they tried, the plan was for another member of their self-help group to bring the "sample" to Hornstein and the rest of the group. Oddly, the donor chose Saran wrap as a receptacle. Peskin recalled, "We opened it up, and it was pretty hard to find! It was pretty ridiculous! It was like an *I Love Lucy* episode. . . . So we got as much of it as we could." Though that attempt (unsurprisingly) failed, Peskin still recalled it as a thrilling and celebratory experience for their group. A whole group of friends stood around Francie taking pictures and talking excitedly. "We said everybody has pictures of their birth, but how many people have pictures of their conception!?"[41]

After about six months of failed attempts with this donor, Hornstein and Peskin decided to seek a second donor. This man was a friend of Suzann Gage, another self-help activist in their group.[42] Again, using fertility consciousness, they waited for the correct timing in Hornstein's cycle. This time, they went to Gage's house to meet the donor. "It was one of the most awkward social experiences I think I've ever had," Hornstein recalled, "standing on Suzann Gage's front porch with this guy we'd never met." After lots of awkward small talk, the group got down to business. "It was a very low-key, low-tech experience. . . . It was very homegrown," Peskin remembered.[43] She, Gage, and Hornstein used a syringe with a cannula attached to the end to insert the sperm, and "it worked! The self-help way."[44]

Hornstein believed that her self-help group's experimentation with self-exam and their familiarity with the anatomy of the cervix made insemination quite simple, and it could for other women as well. Because she had access to medical supplies through the local FWHC, she used a syringe to transfer the semen, but she spoke later with other women who had successfully used other methods. Some employed common household items, such as the now legendary turkey baster. Other women placed sperm inside a diaphragm or a cervical cap and fit the device over their cervix. At least one woman had her donor ejaculate into a condom, which she turned inside out into her vagina.[45] Many women used frequent self-exams in order to determine when they were most fertile, just as women did when using fertility consciousness as a method of contraception. A group of British women who published a pamphlet on self-help donor insemination reported that they received many inquiries from women asking, "Surely it can't be *that* easy?" The group countered that it was, in fact, a simple procedure, as long as a woman was familiar with her body and ovulation cycle.[46]

As this case of donor insemination shows, gynecological self-help activities build on one another. Hornstein used her familiarity with fertility consciousness to get pregnant. Fertility consciousness practitioners used their many experiences with self-exam to help them monitor their fertility. For some, self-help did not end with insemination either, nor did the reliance on a self-help group. Hornstein relied on her self-help group for much of her prenatal care. She also planned to have a home birth. "We were allied with the homebirth movement . . . [and we believed that] with an experienced birth attendant . . . it was safe to have a baby at home." While she labored, there were about ten people there from the health center. Ultimately, complications meant that she had to go to the hospital, where she had a C-section, and the women from the health center went along. When the hospital told her that in order to keep the baby in the room with them over night, they would have to provide and pay for their own private nurses, friends from the health center dressed up in nurses' uniforms and came to stay.[47]

Hornstein and Peskin's group wanted to help others who wanted babies. Women at the Los Angeles FWHC began buying sperm from sperm banks and selling it to women who came to their clinic. Women who came to the clinics to access these services received information and counseling from the staff, and then they had two options: they could either take the sperm home with them, or the clinic staff would help them attempt donor insemination. In general, the clinics preferred that women choose the former and that they have friends or partners help them perform the insemination at home. Another group associated with the Women's Choice Clinic opened the Oakland Sperm Bank in 1984 and became one of the few places in the country where single and lesbian women could buy sperm directly.[48] Some clinics, like the Womancare Feminist Health Center in San Diego, began scheduling workshops to help women find their own donors and learn how to do insemination at home. They did self-exams and practiced squirting water onto their cervixes with needleless syringes.

Self-help activists doing home insemination refused to let doctors, who rarely were willing to inseminate lesbians, until the late 1980s, decide which women were fit to be parents. "We didn't want to medicalize it . . . have to go to a doctor . . . get permission from the medical profession . . . pay for it," Peskin recalled.[49] One study showed that late twentieth-century doctors would sooner inseminate women on welfare, women with contraindications for pregnancy, women infected with STIs, women with criminal records, or women with "less than average" intelligence. Some turned away lesbian women into the 1990s and beyond.[50]

Self-help groups that practiced fertility consciousness and donor insemination found ways to operate entirely outside of the medical system. Though many women in the second half of the twentieth century felt liberated by the availability of birth control methods such the Pill, IUDs, diaphragms, and cervical caps, others saw any form of contraception that forced women to interact with doctors as potentially oppressive. Using fertility consciousness, they found a method of birth control that did not require a doctor's assistance. Similarly, while some women were able to take advantage of physician-aided insemination, other women, particularly single or lesbian women, faced discrimination, exclusion, and disempowerment when they sought to conceive this way. Such women turned to their self-help groups and learned to do inseminations on their own terms, without the aid of a physician.

Self-Help for Older Women

Though a disproportionate number of gynecological self-help activists were young women, under thirty, the movement found support from some older women as well.[51] Some scholars suggest that older women of the 1970s and 1980s were less likely to try self-help because they had grown up in an era when discussing one's body and reproduction was taboo, and self-help simply scandalized them. For these women, self-help was sometimes about "unlearning" to hate or fear their bodies, and shedding feelings they had held for decades. While younger women may also have grown up with similar feelings, scholars suggest that perhaps they were more ingrained in older women. Though self-help appealed widely to younger women, several of the women most often associated with gynecological self-help, including Downer and Rothman, were actually older than thirty when they began practicing self-help.[52]

Often, mothers and daughters discovered self-help together. One woman recalled that, in 1974, she got a surprising gift from her college-age daughter, Rebecca. Rebecca had come home from college excited about self-exam after seeing the mother and daughter team Lolly and Jeanne Hirsch discuss self-help and demonstrate self-exam. Rebecca's mother did a self-examination on herself, and then saw her daughter do one too. They were excited to compare and contrast what they saw. She recalled, "I could distinguish that my vaginal walls had become thinner and smoother, with less configurations than Rebecca's." Some clinics organized self-help groups specifically for mother-daughter pairs.[53]

A brief study of two self-help groups, the Menopause Collective and the October Group, sheds light on how older women used self-help to deal with and even enjoy menopause and aging. Further, examining at these groups gives us a closer look at a perennial problem in feminism: Is it possible for feminists working in small collectives to simultaneously take care of their own needs and offer alternative care for others, or are the two goals intrinsically in conflict?

In the mid-1970s, older women began organizing self-help groups specifically to talk about the realities of menopause and aging. Their work was connected to a larger movement of women that addressed the political and personal issues facing aging women.[54] Some women organized older women's self-help groups from their homes, and others met in groups hosted by local clinics.[55] Most members were women who were approaching or had reached menopause, but they also sometimes included younger women who were interested in menopause and aging.[56] Frustrated with medical interventions in menopause and aging, older women's self-help groups sought ways to live with and even take pleasure in menopause and aging without the aid of doctors or prescription drugs.

Many self-help activists believed that most women's experiences of menopause and aging were shaped by what they called "gynecological imperialism," a system in which "predominantly male gynecologists, profit greedy drug companies, and the federal Food and Drug Administration join forces to practice their disastrous form of sexual politics." They believed that patriarchal institutions led to overprescribing of estrogen, overdiagnosis of osteoporosis, and overuse of hysterectomies. Older women's self-help groups explored alternative ways of dealing with their changing bodies, including taking calcium supplements, altering their diets, and increasing their exercise. They emphasized interacting with the medical system as little as possible. One participant said, "The power of our menopause self-help group movement lies in giving each of us the means to break the medical establishment's stranglehold over our perceptions of and ways to deal with our menopausal experience. We learn that, for most of us, menopause can be a liberating and even . . . a zestful experience!"[57]

The Cambridge Area Menopause Collective, closely associated with the Cambridge WCHC, formed in September 1979 and began meeting monthly. At every meeting, they practiced what some called "internal" self-help where the group members talked about their experiences of aging and discussed strategies for doing so comfortably and without medical intervention.[58] They also frequently facilitated menopause self-help groups for local women who were not part of the Collective. If they chose, women who participated in these local groups could join the Collective once they "graduated" from a four-week self-help group. The Collective also published pamphlets and contributed sections to *Our Bodies, Ourselves*, providing information on how older women could rely on self-help techniques instead of medical or pharmaceutical interventions as they aged. The group saw their outreach work as an alternative to the medical system, a "service for women in the local area."[59]

One of the local groups facilitated by the Menopause Collective, which had begun in October 1979, enjoyed meeting together so much that they decided to continue meeting after their formal four-week session was over. Most of these women also joined the Menopause Collective. The "October Group" met regularly for a few hours a week, and then most of the members adjourned to meet with the rest of the larger Menopause Collective. The Menopause Collective was very task-oriented because they often had to concentrate on organizing the self-help groups they facilitated for the community and on writing and publishing.[60] One member, Kathleen MacPherson, believed that the Menopause Collective functioned like a traditional "male" entity, with agendas, division of labor, and a rigid meeting structure. Because of this rigidity, internal self-help and intimacy often fell by the wayside. "Internal self-help was essentially ignored as we focused on 'spreading the word' about the medicalization of menopause and feminist self-help alternatives," she recalled. Meanwhile, the October Group focused very heavily on doing self-help together, especially dialoguing about their health issues. Rather than following a rigid meeting structure, "anarchy" reigned in their meetings. MacPherson argued that the Menopause Collective was able to survive only because so many of its members also had the October Group as a place to "tak[e] care of our own needs" by practicing self-help. In the Menopause Collective, "we were not practicing what we, as a group, were promoting, namely, self-help."[61] In the October Group, self-help largely took the form of a group discussion of "information, knowledge, experiences, and feelings." Some Collective members who wished to spend more time on internal self-help in Collective meetings felt that the camaraderie and support of self-help in the October Group were as important as the information sharing. On the contrary, other women felt that they could put internal self-help aside and focus on outreach to other women via local self-help groups and writing.[62]

Unsurprisingly, the Menopause Collective also took flak from physicians who disagreed with their stance and tactics. After presenting a workshop for the Bath Brunswick Mental Health Center in Brunswick, Maine, in 1984, MacPherson, who also happened to be a nurse, received a letter from a gynecologist in attendance. He wrote to the board of directors of the Mental Health Center and sent copies of the letter to MacPherson's employer, the dean of the school of nursing where she taught, and to four Maine physicians, saying that her presentation on self-help methods of menopause treatment was "an erroneous one-sided view with marginal half-truths about what the medical profession was doing." MacPherson believed that this doctor was "following a long tradition of gynecologists harassing laywomen who provided healthcare." She replied to the doctor in a letter (also copied to everyone to whom he had sent his letter), saying in rebuttal that even within mainstream medicine, there were differing views on interventions for menopause. She cited several examples from medical professionals, concluding, "My self-help approach is no less legit and less supported by current research in medicine than your approach."[63] MacPherson also questioned this doctor's motives for sharing the letter so widely. She brought both letters to the Collective, which took the opportunity to practice internal self-help in response. They talked about the fears they had as women presenting alternative healthcare. Could they be sued? Lose their jobs? How much time, energy, and money could they devote to dealing with their detractors?[64]

With situations such as this to deal with, the Collective soon discovered that it was difficult to maintain their own self-help activities while simultaneously disseminating information about self-help to other women. If they were going to act completely outside of the medical system, limits on time and energy meant that they had to decide between doing self-help for their own edification and helping other women do self-help. When time constraints eventually led the October Group to disband, its former members felt at a loss and "sorely needed an intimate sharing of experience . . . to create a work-intimacy balance in the Collective."[65] The group firmly believed that with enough support from each other, physician help was largely unnecessary. The trouble was that creating such a support system was a lot of work. For example, in 1983, they committed themselves to distributing 900 packets on self-help menopause information, no small feat in the pre-digital era, and to writing a section of the new edition of *Our Bodies, Ourselves*. Both of these activities included a great deal of original writing from Collective members. Meanwhile, other demands on their time included responding to frequent requests for information from the media (including a number of TV spots and magazine articles), working with other women and groups interested in self-help, and occasionally conducting workshops for interested physicians.[66]

Eventually, they had to decide what their mission truly was: spreading the word about self-help menopause strategies or using self-help to deal with their own health. Some felt that it was crucial to continue sending out information, especially the mailed packets, because rural women in particular might not have any other access to alternative views on menopause; others thought the demands on their time and energy were too great. Some felt that internal self-help was crucial to both the individual women's health and to group cohesion, whereas others viewed self-help discussions as "whining coffee klatches."[67] This issue was so divisive to the group that they even hired two facilitators to help them work it out.[68] Ultimately, the Collective asked the most "task oriented" member to leave; without her present, the group believed that they were better able to balance their time between internal self-help and more limited outreach activities.[69] They cut down on the external Collective activities such as organizing new groups and publishing and began focusing more of their energy on internal self-help.[70] Because the Menopause Collective was so popular and had initiated so many local self-help groups, the National Women's Health Network (NWHN) later formed the Midlife and Older Women's Health Project in order to help older women set up self-help networks to address the issues most salient to their health. They reached out to the Older Women's League, the Gray Panthers, and the Black Women's Health Project for support. Groups continued to focus on issues such as estrogen replacement therapy, hypertension, osteoporosis, menopause, and sexuality. They addressed the way aging women and their bodies were increasingly medicalized and targeted for drug and surgical interactions and discussed tactics for dealing with doctors and healthcare providers. They also focused on coping with the emotional aspects of aging.

Referencing a Federation manual titled *How to Stay Out of the Gynecologist's Office*, an *off our backs* author said, "All one needs is her own speculum and this book (and . . . a self-help clinic) . . . to take care of most problems that arise."[71] As advanced self-help groups discovered, this was an oversimplification. Throughout the 1970s and 1980s, while many self-help practitioners sought creative ways to mold mainstream medicine to their liking, others searched for ways to extricate themselves from that same system. True, laywomen could handle many more aspects of their healthcare than institutional medicine had ever given them credit for. Yet there was often no escaping the very male-dominated institutions they despised. The next chapter also explores how, for women of color and Native American women, this was also an oversimplification, because those concerned with gynecological self-help often had not considered or could not find a way to tackle the complex web of health concerns that many women faced.

5

Looking beyond
the Speculum

Holistic Self-Help

> Why go to a workshop on detecting
> cervical cancer if I don't have the
> self-esteem to even go get the damn
> Pap smear?
> —Loretta Ross

Throughout the late twentieth century, women of color and indigenous women experienced higher rates of illness than their White counterparts. There were many systemic and historical reasons for this injustice. Some lived in areas where it was difficult to access quality healthcare and purchase fresh food because of federal budget cuts to inner-city and rural health centers and cutbacks on food stamps, WIC (the supplemental nutrition program for women, infants, and children), and school lunch programs. Many were disproportionately poor and relied on Medicaid for healthcare; yet many U.S. hospitals admitted only patients referred by a doctor, and many doctors did not accept Medicaid. The federally funded Indian Health Service (IHS), the main provider of medical services on reservations, paid little attention to preventative health services. In immigrant communities, physicians sometimes spoke a different language or were not familiar with cultural or religious norms of their patients. Some were blatantly racist.[1]

Black women, indigenous women, Asian women, and Latinas had participated in gynecological self-help from its inception. Some joined predominantly
White self-help groups, and others created gynecological self-help groups specifically for women of color. A few women of color were clinic founders, dozens worked in feminist clinics as healthworkers, and scores used clinic services.
Yet because the self-help movement's focus remained largely on gynecology
throughout the 1970s, many women of color and indigenous women believed
the movement did not fully consider their needs in its services, strategies, politics, policies, goals, and outreach. Their criticisms of self-help typically fell on
listening ears. In particular, clinic leaders, who were usually White women, dialogued often about how to both expand their clientele and meet the diverse
needs of their clients. Yet other demands on time and energy (particularly confronting anti-abortion activism) along with a persistent belief among many
White, middle-class self-help activists that gynecological self-help really *could*
help all women, meant that sometimes little action happened even as White
feminists heard these criticisms. In the 1980s and 1990s, women of color and
indigenous women began forming self-help-based organizations to address
issues of racial and economic inequality in the women's health and reproductive rights movements; in the process, they developed new uses for and under-
standings of self-help and completely redefined the parameters of the movement.
But it was not merely the de-emphasis on gynecology and self-exam that made
the self-help groups created by women of color and indigenous women unique.
Other self-help groups, such as those for older women, focused a great deal on
dialoguing about emotions and less on physical examinations of their bodies.
Instead, what was unique about the groups created by and for women of color
and indigenous women was their insistence that race and sex were inextricable
and their determination that in order to deal with your physical health, you
have to address your mental health, particularly that which is the result of internalized and institutionalized racism and colonialist structures.

This chapter first explores how the National Black Women's Health Project (NBWHP) developed "holistic" self-help as a way to deal with women's
health problems related to race and racism. It then explores how two other
groups, SisterLove and the Native American Women's Health Education
Resource Center (NAWHERC), adapted holistic self-help strategies to address
the health issues most prevalent in their own communities. SisterLove used self-
help groups to spread awareness about HIV/AIDS and provide support for
infected women.[2] Meanwhile, NAWHERC used self-help to help a reservation
deal with alcohol abuse, fetal alcohol syndrome (FAS), and other related issues.[3]
NBWHP, SisterLove, and NAWHERC self-help groups met a need that both
institutional medicine and predominantly White self-help efforts had not.[4] As
these groups deployed self-help as a holistic method of community healing, they
drew on decades of activism and healthcare traditions by women of color and

indigenous women. Self-help was *critical* to the work of all three of these organizations. Moreover, the work these women did in holistic self-help groups contributed both to an expanding definition of feminism and to the creation of a groundbreaking framework now known as reproductive justice.[5] In the decades after *Roe*, women of color and indigenous women had dramatically expanded the focus of the reproductive rights movement beyond abortion and birth control to include sterilization abuse, other forms of population control, domestic violence, incarceration, childcare, poverty, welfare rights, infant health, and access to basic healthcare.[6] They sought the ability to decide for themselves when to bear and not bear children and the ability to raise children in a wholesome environment.[7] Self-help was a vital piece of developing the reproductive justice framework.

Avery and Allen Develop the Project and the Process

Two activists, Byllye Avery and Lillie Allen, were responsible for developing and fostering holistic, or what they sometimes called "psychological" self-help in the NBWHP. Tracing their paths to the NBWHP helps to explain their goals for psychological self-help, how they developed the practice, and what influence they had on the reproductive justice framework. While Allen developed the psychological self-help method, Avery created a network of Black women to use it. For both women, "health" for the Black community, especially Black women, meant something larger than the physical manifestations of one's body.

Byllye Avery's interest in healthcare came about as a result of her husband's death of a heart attack at age thirty-three. About a decade before, a doctor had told him that his blood pressure was high and encouraged him to exercise and diet. The doctor did not frame his high blood pressure as a life-threatening condition, nor did he follow up with Wesley Avery about changing his diet and exercise habits or give him information on how to make those changes. After her husband's death, Avery began thinking about the importance of understanding family medical history. Wesley's family had a long history of diabetes and cardiovascular diseases, and Avery connected his death to the health habits of the African American community: "how we're reared, what we eat, what foods [we] love, what habits we're into." After his death, she began to think about how important it was for African Americans to be "astute health consumers" and to take care of themselves and each other.[8]

Avery's growing personal interest in healthcare led her to explore a career in reproductive health. In the early 1970s, before *Roe*, while she was working at the Children's Mental Health Unit in Gainesville, Florida, a male colleague asked her and two other women, Margaret Parrish and Judith Levy, to do a small presentation about reproductive rights. As a result of the presentation, local women began to view Avery as an expert, calling her in search of information about where to obtain an abortion. The knowledge that some of these desperate women died because they could not access safe and affordable abortions stuck with Avery.[9] She began participating in consciousness-raising groups made up mostly of White women in Gainesville and read Betty Friedan's *The Feminine Mystique*. "It really opened my eyes, and I could not close them again," she recalled.[10]

Thereafter, working in various jobs at a woman-controlled clinic, a birthing center, and a community college, Avery grew increasingly concerned about the health of Black women. Shortly after *Roe*, she founded and ran the Gainesville Women's Health Center, a feminist clinic that practiced gynecological self-help and offered abortions. Through this work, Avery felt troubled that Black women tended to use the clinic almost exclusively for abortions and did not take advantage of self-help groups and preventative care. In the late 1970s, Avery and three other women from the Gainesville clinic opened Birthplace, a birthing center managed by nurse midwives.[11] Few Black women used the services at Birthplace because they were typically not covered by Medicaid or most insurance plans. In 1980, Avery took a job working for the local community college as a liaison for a job-training program. She spent a lot of time with the Black women students, many of whom were teenagers, and grew worried about their chronic absenteeism. Many had small children at home, and the children's illnesses and activities often kept their mothers from attending school. A number of the students were chronically sick as well, often with diabetes and hypertension. Avery was alarmed at how many of the students had such serious health issues at a young age and did not have access to childcare, transportation, and funds they needed to use medical services. She began to think about ways to expand Black women's access to healthcare.[12]

Around the same time, Avery became involved with the National Women's Health Network (NWHN), a Washington, D.C.–based organization formed in 1975 to monitor federal health agencies and lobby for women's health issues in the federal government.[13] The first person to conduct research on Black women's health for the NWHN, Avery came across a startling statistic: Black women ages eighteen to twenty-five rated themselves in greater distress than similarly aged White women who were officially diagnosed with a mental disorder. "That chilled me," she recalled. "I put my head down and cried."[14] Avery began to think about the "conspiracy of silence" preventing Black women from discussing their psychological distress and recognizing how that distress affected their health. She began organizing the Black Women's Health Project (BWHP) as a division of NWHN in 1981.[15] At the core of Avery's vision for the BWHP (sometimes called "the Project") was a network of Black women's self-help groups, where they could discuss and find ways to cope with their everyday experiences and emotions.[16] "Most of us didn't know how to take care of ourselves because we always took care of everybody else," she remembered. She wanted to create a space for Black women to think and talk about caring for themselves. Avery moved to Atlanta to begin the BWHP and to start planning for a conference on Black women's health. She chose Atlanta because it had a large Black population and because she had a network of activist friends there. Though most of her activist friends were White, many of them had connections to Black women activists, and one friend introduced her to Lillie Allen.[17]

Lillie Allen's interest in self-help came about because of her personal experiences with internalized racism. Allen recalled that when she was an undergraduate at a historically Black college in Florida, other Black students led her to believe she was not good enough to join the "Golden Girl" majorette squad because her hair was the "wrong" texture and her skin was the "wrong" color. In an interview, she reflected that it was ironic that her first memory of being ashamed of her race took place at a historically Black college that sought to foster racial pride. This feeling of shame stuck with her. Years later, while attending graduate school at the University of North Carolina, Chapel Hill, Allen felt her self-doubt reach new heights. As the only African American enrolled in her challenging graduate program, she struggled to contain a constant nagging feeling that everyone else was smarter than she was. Knowing that she wanted to work in health education, Allen began to think more deeply about her own mental and emotional health. She began to ask herself a vital question, "How do I live instead of surviving?" Allen also began to connect these negative feelings she had with racism and to understand that she had internalized many of the racist messages she encountered in her life. She realized that if she wanted to help other people with their health, she would have to begin by dealing with her own.[18]

Allen combined her knowledge of group therapy models with her belief that such programs should engage people politically and began developing a self-help process called "Black and Female," "psychological self-help," or simply, "the process." Allen envisioned Black and Female self-help groups as a place to address systemic and internalized racism and their effects on health. She imagined that each time they met, these self-help groups would pick an issue that affected their health, such as domestic and sexual violence, teenage pregnancy, infant deaths, chronic illness, stress, or self-esteem, and discuss their feelings about it. The idea was that after using self-help to work through their emotions on an issue that affected their health, the women in the group would feel empowered to take action and make changes for themselves and others. "The whole process of Self-Help was supposed to lead to social justice work," health activist (and later Program Director of the Project) Loretta Ross explained. "You get rid of this baggage, this remembered pain, so that you can free up your body, your soul, your spirit to do more work and service to your community."[19]

The newly formed BWHP immediately began using psychological self-help. They formed an organizing committee in Atlanta, a group of about twenty-five Black women, to plan the first National Conference on Black Women's Health

Issues at Spelman College, a historically Black liberal arts college for women in Atlanta. The organizing committee disagreed over what role White women should play at the conference. Avery and a few others wanted to include White women, especially members of the NWHN, since they were funding the conference. Others, including Allen, disagreed. They believed that the work of the conference-goers in addressing their own internalized racism would be difficult enough without having to deal with interracial tensions as well.[20] Allen introduced her version of self-help, "the process," as a way for the group to talk through their emotions surrounding these issues. Allen began by posing a question: How do you feel about White women attending the conference? Then, the women went around the circle and each explained how she felt about the problem.[21] Recalling this first experiment with "the process," Avery noted that it was similar to consciousness-raising from the 1960s and 1970s, but with an added emphasis on "analysis around racism, sexism, and classism."[22] The process created a "trusting atmosphere" so each member of the organizing committee could "talk about her experiences" with internalized oppression "and their effect on her personal choices and decisions." The organizing committee believed that the process helped the entire group to "understand ourselves and each other in different ways." Individual women built "self-esteem" as they divulged and owned their own experiences and decisions. The process also helped the group grow more intimate as they dialogued about how internalized oppression affected their lives. Ultimately, after using the process to work through their feelings as a group, the committee decided that women of any race would be allowed to attend, but that some workshops would be limited to Black women only. Henceforward, because they were so pleased with the outcome, over the two-year period that it took to plan the conference, they began every meeting with the process.[23]

Because they believed that there was a strong connection between health and racialized poverty, the conference organizers worked hard to ensure that the women who attended were not just middle and upper class. They promoted the conference in Black churches, civic organizations, social clubs, colleges and universities, housing projects, nursing homes and senior centers, welfare offices, public health clinics, counseling centers, labor unions, and YWCAs.[24] They sent letters to women, particularly in rural Georgia, within driving distance of the conference, offering them scholarships and transportation.[25] Criteria for receiving a scholarship were an interest in health and an inability to attend without scholarship funding.[26] Ultimately, about a quarter of the conference participants were funded by scholarships.[27] The BWHP hoped that attendees would return to their communities and form hundreds of self-help groups after the conference.[28]

As they considered what type of activities to include in the conference, the committee decided that they needed input from women around the country in order to determine what health issues Black women were interested in addressing. Avery traveled to potential self-help group sites around the South with a slide show about women's health. She also took a "how-to packet" that included health information, reading lists, and information about local and national health agencies. The BWHP helped local women in ten states form their own psychological self-help groups and use the process. Groups often formed around specific health topics, largely based on the expertise or interests of the members. These groups empowered members by helping them build knowledge about health and healthcare while simultaneously giving the BWHP insight into the concerns of local women. The BWHP reported that their most active groups were in rural areas, "where access to health services is a critical problem." After observing the groups in person and talking with members on the telephone, Avery decided that a key ingredient needed for Black women to improve their health was a feeling of empowerment. Many women seemed to believe that they had no control over their own health. She and the conference planning committee discussed how to use the conference to provide women with both new knowledge and a feeling of control.[29]

The First National Conference on Black Women's Health Issues

The first National Conference on Black Women's Health Issues was the first major conference to ever address Black women's health specifically. Avery said that her goal for the conference was "to take care of Black women . . . in a way that nobody has taken care of us before."[30] Here, the process of psychological self-help really cemented as a way for Black women to confront emotions and circumstances that led them down the road to poor health. Original hopes for the conference were for one hundred to two hundred attendees, but as registrations began pouring in, it became clear that the conference would attract closer to two thousand women.[31] On the first day of the conference, women from across the nation arrived in buses and vans, transporting their mothers, sisters, aunts, and grandmothers. One family of women spanning four generations attended, as did Avery's own mother.[32] Avery recalled, "They came with PhDs, MDs, welfare cards, in Mercedes and on crutches, from seven days old to 80 years old—urban, rural, gay, straight."[33] Sixty workshops, films, exhibits, and self-help demonstrations ran throughout the weekend. The conference also featured health screenings, films on natural childbirth, photo exhibits featuring Black women's life cycles, discussions of teen pregnancy, and yoga sessions, all led by Black women healthcare providers and consumers. The most popular programs were the ones that dealt with emotional and psychological health. The conference organizers taped many of the sixty workshops in order to later disseminate them among self-help groups around the nation.[34]

The most popular event at the conference was Allen's psychological self-help workshop, "Black and Female: What Is the Reality?" In the first session, over three hundred women tried to cram into a room designed for fifty people. She had to repeat the workshop every day of the conference in order to satisfy the demand.[35] Women perched on tables and sat on the floor, and many shared a single chair so that they would all fit. At the first session, Allen kicked her shoes off and climbed up on a table. She told the crowd, "We have got to begin moving closer to each other. Get as close as you can. It's past time for holding back."[36] Then she invited the women to begin coming to the front of the room to discuss the struggles of being Black and female.[37]

Slowly, women came forth to tell about childhood rapes, abusive marriages, and health problems.[38] As women told their stories, they laughed and cried. They hugged their old friends and their new "sisters."[39] Allen divided the large group into several smaller ones to continue practicing self-help in this manner. Ross remembered her experience this way: "The next thing you know, you got a room full of Black women crying their hearts out.... As you start peeling back the scabs, it hurts.... Once they dried their tears, it felt like each of us had lost 50 pounds.... You have no idea how heavy the baggage is ... until you get a chance to discharge some of it. All of a sudden, you felt so much emotionally lighter. Really, a catharsis, a really good, soul-cleansing kind of process."[40] For Ross and many of the women at this conference, a self-help workshop about internalized oppression made much more sense than those on gynecological self-help. "Why go to a workshop on detecting cervical cancer if I don't have the self-esteem to even go get the damn Pap smear?" she put it. Using psychological self-help, Black women got to decide for themselves which issues were most crucial to their well-being and to focus first on those.[41] This would later become an important part of the reproductive justice framework. As reproductive justice activists later argued, "While every human being has the same human rights, our intersectional identities require different considerations to achieve reproductive justice."[42]

Disseminating Psychological Self-Help after the Conference

After the conference, the fledgling Black Women's Health Project became the first national health organization devoted strictly to women of color. Both staff and the board of directors of the Project practiced psychological self-help on a regular basis to address how systemic and internalized racism affected their own health.[43] They even held self-help retreats several times a year in the mountains of north Georgia. Group leaders from around the country gathered with the staff from the Atlanta office and spent the weekend doing psychological self-help.[44]

The BWHP saw that gynecological self-help groups had successfully created awareness around reproductive health issues, and they wanted to create a similar awareness around health issues affected by race or exacerbated by racism.[45] As the Project's literature explained, "facilitators of... [gynecological] self-help groups did not consider, or were unable to respond to, the difficulties experience[d] by Black women."[46] The Project developed its own self-help groups as a direct "response to the limitations of this... [gynecological] self-help movement."[47] In addition, BWHP leaders saw their psychological self-help groups as a continuation of the kinds of self-improvement and community uplift projects Black women had been involved with for many decades.[48] In 1984, the BWHP became the National Black Women's Health Project (NBWHP) and organized as a separate entity from the predominantly White NWHN.[49] They set up a national headquarters in Atlanta in a sixteen-room robin's-egg blue clapboard house on two and a half acres. They filled the headquarters with plush sofas and covered the walls in tapestries, paintings, and conference posters and threw their energy into forming psychological self-help groups across the nation.[50]

Psychological self-help groups began by asking, "What health problems are we experiencing?" and "What do we need to do to take charge of our lives?" Because of their high rates of poverty, Black women were often at an increased risk of hypertension, heart disease, diabetes, kidney disease, and obesity. Since they frequently lacked quality healthcare, Black women also had much higher rates of death from diseases such as cancer. Black infant mortality rates were double the rates for White infants. The NBWHP estimated that all of these factors, combined with the stress of economic hardships, left more than half of Black women in psychological distress. Their goal was to use self-help groups to embolden Black women to tackle these race-related health problems.[51] Most importantly, they wanted to view health holistically, tackling problems at their roots. Since Black women were more likely to suffer from stress-related illnesses, the NBWHP thought that it was important to tackle sources of stress (which were often related to money, racism, and feelings of self-worth) at the source. They believed that self-help groups could help Black women equip themselves with tools to confront the emotions that often led them down the road to poor health.

Some women who had been involved in gynecological self-help before the conference had to decide whether to embrace psychological self-help or mostly stick with gynecological self-help. For example, the Black Women's Self-Help Collective, which had formed in the early 1980s specifically to bring cervical self-exam to their D.C. community, attended the conference as a group, and several members went to Allen's Black and Female Workshop. After the conference, this group debated whether to continue their work with gynecological self-help or to form a chapter of the National Black Women's Health Project and focus on psychological self-help. They chose the latter, because they wanted to be part of a larger network of Black women and to expand their focus beyond gynecology. Thereafter, this group did not completely ignore gynecology; instead they integrated it into a more holistic view of health. Similarly, the larger NBWHP saw gynecological self-help strategies such as cervical self-exam as one of many self-help techniques available to them.[52] This mind-set was typical of many Black feminists of the era. Rather than rejecting the strategies and goals of mainstream feminism, they tended to expand upon them, taking an "intersectional" view of feminism and paying attention to how race, gender, and class together influenced a woman's experiences. These attitudes have been enormously influential on more recent modes of feminism as well.

By the late 1980s, the NBWHP's network of self-help groups had expanded greatly. At first, the Project mostly consisted of a few loosely connected self-help groups in large cities such as Atlanta, Philadelphia, and New York. Within five years after the conference, there were chapters in twenty-two states. In 1989 Avery won a MacArthur Fellowship, or "Genius Grant," an annual award of $500,000.[53] As a result of the publicity she received from the award, membership in the NBWHP exploded. Project staff described the phone ringing constantly for months as women from all over the nation sought information about starting their own chapters.[54] Ross, who had just accepted a job as director, began hiring regional directors to help form chapters and set to work writing a self-help manual.[55] The NBWHP offered assistance to local dues-paying chapters over the phone, visited the groups in person, and wrote how-to guides for local chapters to use. They kept careful track of the local chapters, who reported their activities frequently in order to maintain membership status. The national office in Atlanta also helped local groups raise funds, manage their finances, and coordinate media attention. The NBWHP also facilitated connections among local chapters by holding regional and national meetings, retreats, and training sessions. Meanwhile, the leaders continued to practice self-help among themselves.[56]

The structure of an NBWHP self-help group meeting was fairly rigid. Groups had rotating facilitators whose job it was to ask a question to get the discussion started.[57] Ross recalled that these questions could include anything from "What went on with your week that makes you feel good?" to "What would you have liked to accomplish in your life that you haven't had a chance to do?" to "When have you felt someone hurt you?" Many groups had a time limit in which each person had a chance to respond. Others allowed participants to talk for as long as they felt comfortable. Typically, responding to another person's story with questions or thoughts was taboo, "because people's stories are owned by the people who are telling the stories. So their stories aren't there for your curiosity or your edification or for you to ask them questions so that you can find out more or learn more," noted Ross.[58] The NBWHP was adamant that members should not view self-help groups as a form of group ther-apy or as a place to air grievances or get advice. Avery said that self-help groups were not an appropriate place to say, "Sister, go get your Pap smear." Instead, self-help groups were a place for women to listen to each other's stories. Mem-bers should ask, "Sister ... what's on top for you?" If keeping up with bills or low self-esteem were the issues "on top" for a woman, then the group's role was to help her come to terms with those issues. The NBWHP believed that address-ing what was "on top" was the only way for a woman to improve her overall health.[59]

One major goal of the NBWHP was to reach low-income women with limited access to healthcare.[60] Eighteen NBWHP-affiliated self-help groups formed in several public housing developments around Atlanta. In 1988, to further support these groups, the NBWHP founded the Center for Black Women's Wellness (CBWW), a community-based center in Mechanicsville (near Atlanta) to provide a place for poor local women to get medical screen-ings, learn job skills, and access resources, particularly for pregnancy. The CBWW hosted programs for adults and teens to gather and talk about sexu-ality, provided tutoring and career counseling, and offered help for young women to obtain their GED. The CBWW was an extension of self-help groups. For these women, school and jobs were "on top." In order to be healthy, young women needed access to basic education and career services.[61] Considering health holistically meant that a woman could not think about her physical health until these needs were met.

After publishing hundreds of pamphlets and newsletters on self-help in the 1980s, in the early 1990s the NBWHP began to publish books to reach women who may not have been able to attend an in-person self-help group.[62] The Proj-ect sponsored member Linda Villarosa's *Body and Soul: The Black Women's Guide to Physical Health and Emotional Well-Being*, a book that sought to "end the damaging conspiracy of silence about the realities of Black women's lives."[63] Having spent five years as the health editor of *Essence* magazine, Villarosa believed that "Black women were hungry for health information. . . . Any time we did a story about health, we'd get so many, many calls and letters, and if we listed a resource name and number that person was just overwhelmed."[64] Yet when Villarosa first took her idea for *Body and Soul*, a self-help guide by and for Black women, to a publisher in 1986, the publisher rejected it. Everyone she approached at first seemed skeptical about whether "Black people buy books."[65] Ultimately, in 1994, Harper Collins agreed to publish the book, which it mar-keted as "the first self-help book for Black women." The book had dozens of contributors: sixteen authors, four doctors, sixty first-person storytellers, a team of consultants from NBWHP, and a foreword by Angela Davis and June Jor-dan.[66] According to Villarosa, some of the contributors shared their stories not only to help other women, but to help themselves.[67] The title, *Body and Soul*, was an apt summary of the Project's overall philosophy; the book addressed physical and emotional health simultaneously. Villarosa believed that physicians as well as most books on health failed to address "the whole person." For example, she said, "The doctor treats the high blood pressure, but pays little attention to what's driving the pressure up in the first place."[68] The book encouraged women to take action to improve both the healthcare system and their individual health. "It's about learning to stand up for yourself in the healthcare system, and most importantly about self-esteem. If you really love yourself, then you'll take care of yourself," Villarosa told the *Orange County Register*. There was also an entire chapter on dealing with doctors. As one reviewer said, "You may not be able to find a Black woman doctor but at least you can learn to talk to the white male doctors you will probably be faced with."[69] The book also explored a variety of "alternative" methods of healing, including acupuncture, aromatherapy, and homeopathy. Much of the focus was on diet and exercise, "not just because it will help you live longer, but because you'll feel better," said Villarosa. The book offered women a chance to learn about their bodies. It also included a liberal dose of lessons about the shortcomings of institutional medicine and encouraged women to take their health into their own hands.[70]

Sometimes "the process" bred conflict. Allen saw self-help as an essential part of the organization's decision-making process.[71] However, there were some women who did not want to participate because they saw it as "cultish" and "touchy-feely." Some members thought this conflict had a class element. Ross recalled that the "professional, health-oriented women" were not interested in talking about feelings and pain. "They wanted to talk about how to get more Black women to get Pap smears. Lillie wanted to talk about why Black women who knew they needed Pap smears weren't getting them."[72] Sources tell conflicting stories about how the leadership of the NBWHP divided, but disagreements over self-help certainly contributed to what became a split between Avery and Allen.[73] Because she held a leadership position in the NBWHP, Avery believed that it was inappropriate for her to share certain aspects of her life when doing self-help with other staff.[74] She believed that some things were too personal to tell her co-workers. One major tenet of NBWHP self-help was that group members must never reveal to others what they had learned about another member in a self-help session. Avery stopped doing self-help when another woman told a larger group something Avery had said in a self-help session.[75] Despite these problems, Allen continued to insist that self-help was the organization's life and soul and that it was a huge misstep for a leader to opt out.[76] Perhaps knowing that the conflict between herself and Avery was about to come to a head, Allen copyrighted the phrase "Black and Female: What Is the Reality?" in 1988.[77] Avery was livid. She felt that the concept belonged to the entire NBWHP.[78] Tensions between the two sides grew heated. Some felt that it made more financial sense for the organization to shift its focus away from self-help. They thought it would be easier to get funding to do policy work to improve Black women's health than to support self-help organizing.[79]

In 1990, after extensive attempts at conflict resolution, the Project decided that self-help would no longer be its major focus.[80] They opened a public education and policy office in Washington, D.C. and eventually moved their headquarters there. Allen left the Project. In 2002, the Project changed its name to the Black Women's Health Imperative (BWHI). Today, the BWHI focuses on policy rather than grassroots self-help. A few self-help local chapters still exist, and they do so largely independently of the BWHI.[81] Yet self-help did not disappear from women of color's health organizations. Instead, it lived on in groups that formed after the Project, including both SisterLove and NAWHERC. The BWHI considers "the self-help legacy as its most significant contribution to the movement." The remainder of this chapter examines how these two groups live out this legacy.[82]

SisterLove

Dazon Dixon Diallo was lucky enough to attend the First Conference on Black Women's Health in 1983 because she was a student at Spelman at the time. Afterward, she began thinking not only about Black women's health, but also about the particular needs of the community around her campus. Dixon Diallo recalled, "If I had to walk from Spelman to the West End and came across . . . young women who were pregnant, pushing buggies, what would I be able to do about that?" When she began looking for a job the next year, she found one as a healthworker at the Atlanta FWHC, where she was both the youngest member of staff and the only woman of color.[83]

Dixon Diallo's six-year stint (1984–1989) at the Atlanta FWHC coincided with the height of the HIV/AIDS crisis in the United States.[84] Though the mysterious virus may have existed in the United States for perhaps as much as two decades prior, in 1981, U.S. physicians began to pay a lot of attention when a group of previously healthy gay men in New York and California suddenly fell ill. Panic over the disease spread quickly because many people died within weeks of a diagnosis.[85] The Centers for Disease Control (CDC) designated HIV/AIDS an epidemic and said that the number of infected people so far was likely just "the tip of the iceberg."[86] Lack of understanding about how it spread led to heightened anxieties about homosexuality.[87] The media even briefly referred to the disease as "gay related immune deficiency" or "GRID."[88] By 1983, however, when several women who had male partners with HIV/AIDS contracted it as well, it became clear that heterosexual sex could also spread the disease. By the end of that year, over three thousand cases of AIDS had been reported in the United States, and nearly thirteen hundred of that number had died. The original panic over the disease's connection to gay White men meant that few physicians or organizations paid attention to other populations with high incidences of infection.[89]

Dixon Diallo quickly realized that HIV/AIDS prevention posed special problems for women of color and poor women. They were more likely to lack health insurance and access to preventative medical care.[90] Poor women were statistically less likely to be educated about how to prevent sexually transmitted infections or to seek help when they notice symptoms.[91] Moreover, HIV transmission is also linked to domestic violence. For example, sexual abusers (who might be infected) were unlikely to wear condoms. Women of color were more likely to experience and less likely to report domestic violence because of fears of discrimination from social service agencies.[92] In the early 1980s, Black women in Georgia were thirteen times more likely to get HIV than their White counterparts, and it was the fifth leading cause of death among Black women in the state.[93]

As the AIDS epidemic intensified, the Atlanta FWHC began offering more testing and education for HIV/AIDS. When women in Atlanta began inundating a local organization that mostly served gay men with AIDS, that organization reached out to the FWHC in hopes of collaboration, since they were overwhelmed by the volume of women's calls and were less sure about how to help women with the disease.[94] In 1987, Dixon Diallo helped create the FWHC's Women with AIDS Partnership Project (WAPP), which held "Do It Safe Parties" in public housing projects, drug treatment programs, transitional halfway settings after prison release, battered women's shelters, and homeless shelters. At these "parties," women shared stories as a group and educated themselves about safe sex and HIV/AIDS prevention. They also discussed the disproportionate impact of HIV/AIDS on socioeconomically disadvantaged women and dialogued about the political implications of the epidemic. The FWHC tried to model these "parties" after self-help groups. They were intended as a space for women to share information and learn to either prevent HIV or manage their disease if they already had it.[95]

Yet Dixon Diallo felt that the FWHC did not adequately connect its reproductive health services with HIV/AIDS prevention, and she saw this as a symptom of the gulf between Black and White women's health activism. "Because HIV and AIDS at that time was more indicative of poor women and women who were active drug users . . . those issues did not necessarily connect for folks who were leading the movement for equality for women or for equal pay or for access to abortion," she recalled. Dixon Diallo began to understand that "this was going to be a Black woman's issue."[96] HIV/AIDS was not "on the radar" of the White middle-class feminists running the FWHC. "And that's what it felt like . . . for those of us women of color in the community: that AIDS is not their issue, but it is ours, and we'd better do something about it."[97]

Dixon Diallo also recognized a financial logic behind why the clinic did not prioritize HIV/AIDS awareness. As she put it, "From a very practical standpoint, when you are providing abortions, you already have a heavy cross to bear." In the late 1980s, the Democratic National Convention took place in Atlanta, and alongside this event, the powerhouse anti-abortion group Operation Rescue began holding clinics around the city "under siege." This took a great toll on the energy and finances of the FWHC, so anything that did not generate much revenue (such as HIV/AIDS services) had to go.[98]

When the funding for HIV/AIDS work at the FWHC disappeared, Dixon Diallo had to decide what to do next.[99] In 1989, she left the FWHC with a $2,500 grant from the Fund for Southern Communities (and unemployment benefits) and started a nonprofit called SisterLove, an organization devoted to HIV/AIDS prevention and education, particularly for women at risk of or already living with HIV/AIDS.[100] SisterLove originally focused its efforts around Atlanta and targeted "predominantly black women, of child-bearing age, socio-economically disadvantaged, with less than a high school education." Dixon Diallo wanted to find at least one hundred women who were HIV positive and educate them and their families and partners about how the disease was spread as well as coordinate social services and healthcare for the infected women. Dixon Diallo quickly saw that many women of color and poor women knew that HIV/AIDS was a "contagious disease that kills," but their knowledge usually ended there. Many women continued to see AIDS as a disease that predominantly affected gay White men and did not understand the risks for women and for people in heterosexual relationships or the Black community in general.[101] In Georgia, about 25 percent of the people diagnosed with HIV/AIDS were women, and a shocking 84 percent of those women were Black.[102] Because they were less likely to seek treatment, Black men and women died *six* times faster than White men and women.[103] Women who contracted HIV often felt alone and bewildered. Juanita Williams, who found SisterLove after she was diagnosed with HIV in 1989, recalled, "I definitely felt like I was the only woman [with the disease]. There was no place to go and no one to talk to."[104]

Dixon Diallo believed that SisterLove needed to tackle HIV/AIDS as a social issue, not just a medical one. That is, they would have to consider the ways the conditions of a person's life affected her likelihood of contracting HIV/AIDS and her ability to manage it. For example, "a poor intravenous drug user who is depending on others for a fix, cannot afford her own clean needles, and is forced to share needles with others runs a higher risk of being infected with HIV than does someone who does not share syringes for intravenous drugs."[105] Understanding how these intersecting oppressions affected both risk factors and treatment was paramount if Black women were to deal with the mounting HIV/AIDS crisis.

SisterLove used self-help to approach HIV/AIDS prevention and management in a sex positive way. They wanted people to be able to have a "safe and enjoyable sex life, regardless of HIV status."[106] This was a dramatically different standpoint than that of many other Black institutions that were concerned with HIV/AIDS, particularly male-led Black churches, which tended to encourage abstinence.[107] Dixon Diallo befriended Byllye Avery, who helped her think about how to start and run the organization. She soon discovered that she needed to provide a space for more than education and awareness. She needed to find a way for women to support each other. Self-help was the solution. Instead of passively receiving information about HIV/AIDS, SisterLove groups worked together to educate themselves about preventing or living with HIV/AIDS.[108]

SisterLove leaders (usually about four women) also did self-help among themselves using a process much like the one the Project developed. These leader-level groups were especially helpful after challenging self-help groups with HIV positive women. These leader-level self-help groups were also designed to think about how to help women create change. Dixon Diallo gave this example: "If we were holding a . . . self-help session and it seemed like everybody in the room was having a problem with being treated badly in the homes where they were living . . . when we came back together to debrief ourselves from those self-help sessions and have our own self-help, we would come to our own solutions about how to help." In one case, in 1992, this led SisterLove to create a housing program; LoveHouse was a transitional housing facility for HIV positive women.[109] The residents attended weekly support meetings and education workshops.[110]

As with the Project, Dixon Diallo also wanted to use self-help to empower women to help others. SisterLove began working with HIV positive women to help them "become leaders . . . in their own communities." Some founded their own organizations and became members on boards of directors, national spokespersons for HIV/AIDS education, and international members of UN-level coalitions and organizations.[111]

Dixon Diallo felt it was crucial for women in SisterLove self-help groups to "go back into why this was even a threat to us in the first place." Group members talked about why they were at a disproportionately high risk for this disease in the first place. They also had to tease out what risk factors they could control themselves. Dixon Diallo recalled that it was "the same stuff that we had . . . learned in self-help through the National Black Women's Health Project. It was the walking wounded stuff, you know? It was the experiences, the traumas, the things that we've gone through in our lives that drive us to the decisions, or the non-decisions."[112] SisterLove groups talked about systemic and internalized oppressions that had prevented them from seeking care or learning about prevention. Then they worked on strategies to live happy and fulfilling lives as HIV positive people. In the late 1980s, many people believed that an HIV diagnosis was a death sentence. Families disowned members who contracted HIV, and people refused to eat near or share a bathroom with an infected person. People lost their jobs, marriages, children, and friends. People who were HIV positive had extremely elevated rates of depression and suicide, especially right after they received a diagnosis. SisterLove self-help groups helped women deal with all of these losses, make new friends, and even regain old friends and family members. Reflecting on the importance of SisterLove groups later, Loretta Ross said that she believed that for some women, these self-help groups were literally lifesaving.[113]

Self-Help at the Native American Women's Health Education Resource Center

In the late 1980s, Charon Asetoyer, a Comanche Indian from San Jose, California, with a background in health education and intercultural management, brought self-help to her community on the Yankton Sioux Reservation in South Dakota. Though she personally identified as a feminist, Asetoyer, like many other women of color and indigenous women, thought that mainstream feminism did not accurately reflect the diversity of women in the movement. "For Indigenous feminists, it did not make sense to separate women's issues from larger community issues," she said.[114] In order to address the myriad difficulties that plagued indigenous women and their communities, Asetoyer developed a new self-help approach that took indigenous traditions and spirituality into account.

Native Americans on South Dakota reservations faced myriad health concerns. In South Dakota, over half of all domestic violence cases occurred in Native American households, though Native Americans made up less than 7 percent of the population. Seventy-five percent of Yankton Sioux Reservation residents over forty had diabetes. Eighty-five percent of the Native American adults on the reservation were unemployed. Only about a third of indigenous women in the state received regular prenatal care. The infant mortality rate in South Dakota was on the rise; there were 28.8 deaths per 1,000 births (more than double the national average). Three percent of all children on the reservation were born with fetal alcohol syndrome.[115]

At the heart of many feminist self-help efforts was a desire to prevent health problems before they occur; this was certainly the case with Asetoyer's work. Native Americans in the United States still felt the effects of exploitation by European and American settlers spreading across the continent, seizing land, and wreaking havoc on Native civilizations. Asetoyer recognized that many of the health issues her community faced grew in part out of long-term effects of colonialism, including poor healthcare and alcohol abuse. In the mid-1980s, over 90 percent of the Yankton Sioux Reservation population relied for health-care on the federally funded Indian Health Service (IHS), which existed as a result of treaty obligations that required the U.S. government to provide health-care on reservations.[116] Many people did not feel a sense of confidentiality and security when dealing with the federally funded IHS, so they were hesitant to take advantage of its services. Women were often especially loath to use IHS services for reproductive care, because they resented the intrusion of the federal government into practices long controlled by women.[117] Among Plains tribes, older women had traditionally delivered children, then mentored girls through puberty and into adulthood. When those older women grew too old to care for themselves, the children they had delivered and mentored took care of them. When the IHS took over healthcare on reservations in the mid-twentieth century, many elderly women were pushed out of their role as mid-wives and purveyors of Native women's health traditions and threatened with legal penalties if they failed to comply. This disruption in traditional care left many Native women without healthcare they could trust.[118] Asetoyer also believed that when the IHS did focus on preventative measures, their efforts were misguided. She offered this example: In a discussion about preventing fetal alcohol syndrome, one IHS doctor suggested prescribing Depo-Provera, an injectable form of birth control, to alcoholic women. Yet there was "no talk . . . of trying to help a woman with her chemical dependency."[119] Like Avery and Allen, Asetoyer believed that many women in her community had "internalized barriers," including a lack of self-esteem, because of lifelong experiences of racism and colonialism. Recognizing that these barriers were negatively affecting Native American women's overall health, she began looking for a way to address them.[120]

Asetoyer and her husband helped start an organization called the Native American Community Board (NACB) on the Yankton Sioux Reservation in Lake Andes, South Dakota. The organization, founded in 1986, began developing programs to address Native people's health, education, land and water rights, and economic development issues.[121] Asetoyer quickly honed in on fetal alcohol syndrome as an issue of high importance because of its prevalence on her reservation and because the IHS was doing so little to combat it.[122] She believed that the IHS often "wrote off" women who were chemically dependent, many of whom were unaware of the effects of drinking while pregnant.[123] Many scholars and activists contend that high levels of alcoholism among Native Americans was the result of what feminist theorist M. Annette Jaimes called "colonially induced despair," a feeling of both individual and collective hopelessness as a result of European colonization. Instead of helping women deal with the root causes of alcohol abuse, the IHS found short-term solutions.[124] Because she believed that it was impossible to confront FAS without tackling all of the related health and education issues indigenous mothers faced,

Asetoyer wanted a place where women could work on all of these problems together.[125] If the IHS was not going to confront the root causes, women would have to "take the initiative" themselves and practice self-help methods of treatment and prevention. "The responsibility of protecting and providing for our nation falls right into our hands, as grandmothers, mothers, aunties, and sisters," she said.[126] Asetoyer began to think about buying a small house on the reservation and opening a self-help-based center to address local women's health issues. She wanted a place equipped with a kitchen for nutrition classes and a yard for children to play in.[127]

Though the impetus to create a self-help-based center came from local concerns, Asetoyer's connections to a wider network of women's health and self-help activists influenced her as well. As she thought about opening a center, Asetoyer began attending health conferences and meetings and soon met other influential members of the women's health and self-help movements. In the mid-1980s, she met Byllye Avery through a mutual friend and visited the NBWHP headquarters in Atlanta.[128] In 1988, she also joined the board of the NWHN and attended a national conference, where she met National Latina Health Organization (NLHO) founder Luz Martinez. Martinez and the NLHO had been working on developing self-help-based programs for Latinas since 1986.[129] Asetoyer told Martinez about her idea for a Native American women's center. Martinez loved the idea and encouraged her to reach out to other women at the conference for monetary support. "Go for it," she told her. "I won't let you leave until you let these women know. They can help. They believe in helping women!" When Asetoyer made an announcement about the house at lunch, Avery was the first to take out her checkbook. Word spread around the conference about Asetoyer's idea, and before it ended, she had collected over $2,000 toward the house. That same year, with support from the NACB, Asetoyer opened the Native American Women's Health Education Resource Center.[130]

Self-help was at the core of all of NAWHERC's early efforts. As their mission statement read, NAWHERC was founded "based on a self-help philosophy, promoting individual and group involvement in the betterment of our lives as Native Americans."[131] Scholars have largely overlooked NAWHERC's self-help philosophy, and a few have argued that they did not practice self-help at all. In fact, the organization developed a hybrid mix of self-help activities. NAWHERC employed elements of psychological self-help, gynecological self-help, and traditional Native American processes.[132]

For NAWHERC, self-help involved demystifying mainstream healthcare while leaving room for culturally appropriate, traditional, woman-controlled methods as well.[133] One way that they facilitated this goal was by working to capture and re-create traditional elements of healing. NAWHERC organized self-help groups where older women in the community could talk to younger women. The elder women often spoke about how, traditionally, Native women had the power to "determine the size of their families." They told stories of the "various techniques and . . . medicines to terminate a pregnancy" that had long been known to their community. In response, at many such groups, the other women in the group quickly begin to tell their own stories, especially about abortion and childbirth. Other voices chimed in, emphasizing a desire to "live and raise [their] famil[ies] free of violence, to have housing, to have food, to have clean water, clean air," and pointing out the connections between the loss of control over their reproductive selves and colonialism.[134] Asetoyer said, "Self-help for us is . . . to have that knowledge and power so that we know what to do and when to do it and not just leave everything up to the Indian Health Service and the physicians that were being driven . . . [by] these oppressive policies that were violating our human rights."[135] The self-help format resonated with many women, because passing information from older women to younger ones in this way honored a centuries-old oral tradition of learning through storytelling. Though self-help was often intergenerational, for NAWHERC this was a key element, one they could not do without.[136] Their self-help groups put the issues they faced in the context of internalized oppression while simultaneously connecting their healing to a spiritual element. NAWHERC sometimes called self-help groups "roundtables" or "talking circles" and took opportunities to say "thank you to the creator." This holistic process integrated mental, physical, and spiritual healing.[137] The roundtable format, much like other self-help group formats, emphasized that "all community members are experts through their life experiences and have the necessary information and solutions to address their concerns." Often, at the end of a roundtable, the participants worked together to come up with a solution to individual or community problems.[138] They frequently published reports of the roundtable and made them available to the public. Sometimes the goal was to disseminate information, and sometimes it was to put pressure on the IHS to change its policies, for example, by providing more prenatal care on the reservation and not pushing Depo-Provera on women with contraindications.[139] NAWHERC also hired a full-time employee whose primary duties revolved around developing self-help activities to prevent FAS. She set up and monitored self-help groups, where women living on the reservation talked about alcoholism and health. Understanding the need to address these issues holistically, NAWHERC expanded its focus to issues related to alcoholism and FAS and brought other services to the reservation, all based on a self-help philosophy. Their goal was to create a place for women to "organize around issues of concern, social change, and consciousness raising activities." Because they believed that alcohol abuse was often related to employment and personal relationships, NAWHERC also offered self-help groups for women experiencing domestic abuse and skill-building classes for both adults and children, especially around computer education.[140]

In order to confront FAS in the context of reproductive justice, NAWHERC believed it was important to both help women understand their own bodies and simultaneously expose the IHS's failings.[141] NAWHERC also published and disseminated literature on alcoholism and FAS, encouraging women on the reservation and beyond to learn about these conditions and take action for themselves. They developed literature that was both lay-friendly (not laden with medical jargon) and relevant to indigenous women.[142] To demystify reproductive care and women's bodies, they published pamphlets such as *A Girl's Guide to Menstruation, A Young Woman's Guide to Pap Smears*, and *Know the Facts about Menstruation and Hormone Replacement Therapy.* NAWHERC also held seminars on aspects of reproductive health ranging from teenage pregnancy and AIDS to the socioeconomics of single parenting. Meanwhile, they worked to document and publicize the IHS's violations of Native women's rights, especially around gynecology and reproduction. The idea was that if women understood their own bodies and were aware of IHS practices, they could make informed choices about their own healthcare.[143]

NAWHERC quickly turned its focus beyond the Yankton Sioux Reservation, and in 1990 it helped organize the Empowerment through Dialogue: Native American Women and Reproductive Rights Conference at Pierre, South Dakota, a gathering that emphasized self-help solutions to reproductive health problems. Women representing eleven tribes in North and South Dakota met to talk about traditional Native American methods of abortion and childbirth rituals, many of which had been disrupted by colonialism and forced assimilation. Many conference attendees advocated a return to these methods as a way for indigenous women to regain control over their reproduction. Attendees also discussed the poor state of prenatal care on reservations. NAWHERC asked a group of women from a woman-controlled clinic to demonstrate self-exam at the conference. Asetoyer recalled that the young women in particular were especially eager to try self-exam and that they quickly connected this skill with increased control and ownership over their bodies.[144]

Because alcoholism often correlated with diabetes, in 1991 NAWHERC also created self-help groups for the reservation's diabetic population. In small self-help groups, participants came together to learn skills to manage the disease in order to reduce the secondary complications of diabetes (such as blindness and heart disease). Each group met for ten one-hour sessions over a period of five weeks. They discussed the reasons behind the high rates of diabetes in the community, especially the ready availability of high-sodium and high-fat foods. They learned to read blood glucose (or blood sugar) levels, maintained weight charts, and learned about stress management techniques, as well as developing good exercise and nutrition habits. Participants dialogued about the connection between diabetes and alcohol and talked about how the disease affected them personally. They did research to find exercises that were possible for people who were already overweight. To determine how well self-help methods were working in these groups, NAWHERC conducted a study of the participants' blood sugar levels. (Individuals with diabetes have higher than average blood sugar levels.) NAWHERC found that when compared to a control group who did not participate in self-help groups, participants drastically decreased their blood sugar level. They also found that as much as a year after the study, participants continued to monitor their own levels and consistently kept them lower. As with groups that dealt with FAS, these diabetes groups filled a void that the IHS left open.[145]

"Why go to a workshop on detecting cervical cancer if I don't have the self-esteem to even go get the damn Pap smear?" self-help activist Loretta Ross posited. In the 1980s and 1990s, African American and indigenous women searched for ways to end the "conspiracy of silence" surrounding their health struggles and developed self-help practices to address issues most salient in their communities. These groups created an entirely new kind of self-help based on what was "on top" for their communities. Avery, Allen, Dixon Diallo, and Asetoyer believed that one had to look "beyond the speculum," beyond a woman's reproductive system, beyond even her body.

Because of their attention to holistic health, the NBWHP, SisterLove, and NAWHERC broadened the focus of the self-help movement to include issues well beyond gynecology. In doing so, they fundamentally reshaped the movement. Further, they contributed to an expanding definition of feminism, bringing not only an awareness of the intersectionality of women's health experiences, but also the tools with which women could deal with those realities of their lives that were shaped by interlocking oppressions. Through these projects, it is easy to see that the parameters of "self-help," "feminism," and even "women's health" grew both larger and murkier over time. Women of color and indigenous feminists also demonstrated that the self-help movement needed to be broader than reproductive rights. In order to truly address the needs of all women, the self-help movement had to consider reproductive *justice*. As Dixon Diallo put it, self-help was the "track" upon which the "train" of organizations that did reproductive justice work rolled. It helped women stick together when their interests diverged or the burden of activism became too heavy. It connected women to each other and to themselves. "Reproductive justice cannot be achieved without self-help," she told Ross. "If we don't have a continued way to stay at the table when things get hard, eventually, we will all get up from that table."[146]

6

Reintroducing Menstrual Extraction

Self-Help Abortion after *Roe*

> Twenty years ago, saying we were going
> to do our own abortions was like saying
> we were going to build our own nuclear
> bombs. Today, we know we can do it
> ourselves.
> —Carol Downer

In spite of the growing parameters of the self-help movement in the 1980s, abortion remained a central focus for many self-help activists, especially middle-class White women. This was particularly evident in the changing and growing activism surrounding menstrual extraction. In the late 1980s and early 1990s, because of increased anti-abortion activism and new legislation, women around the nation began to fear that abortions in clinics and hospitals might soon become unavailable. Some self-help activists, led by the Federation of Feminist Women's Health Centers (the Federation), responded by endorsing menstrual extraction as a self-help method of abortion. Their advocacy was conspicuously different from early 1970s rhetoric, which tended to carefully avoid designating menstrual extraction as an abortion technique. In the 1980s and 1990s, these self-help activists felt that it was not only vital to master menstrual extraction as an abortion method but also to publicly promote it as such.

This exploration of self-help activists' promotion and practice of menstrual extraction in the late 1980s and early 1990s complicates most scholarly accounts of the women's health movement, which associate the practice of menstrual extraction with the years before *Roe v. Wade*. After 1973, these studies suggest, menstrual extraction fell out of favor, replaced by methods of abortion performed by doctors.[1] In fact, from 1973 through the late 1980s, even as they explored other uses for self-help, women in "advanced" groups around the United States continued to practice the technique and to disseminate information about it. Typically, they flew under the radar, attracting little attention from the mainstream media (except for one case in 1978 discussed briefly in this chapter). The situation changed in 1988, a moment when anti-abortion protest groups increasingly tried to restrict women's access to abortion clinics and new laws challenged and chipped away at *Roe*. In response, feminist health activists introduced menstrual extraction to wider audiences and presented this technique explicitly as a method of pregnancy termination—what they called "early abortion." While touring the country, seeking media attention, and publishing information on menstrual extraction, they emphasized that making abortion illegal would not make it go away.[2]

The revival of menstrual extraction was a proactive strategy used by self-help activists to try to preserve abortion rights in the face of an onslaught of threats from anti-abortion activists and the government. Self-help had always blurred the lines between groups of feminists, and it even complicates our understanding of who was a "mainstream" feminist. NOW has long been seen as the bastion of mainstream and liberal feminism. Yet, in the late 1980s and early 1990s, this "mainstream" organization once again cooperated with radical, underground actions designed specifically to subvert the law if abortion were to become illegal.[3]

But what of holistic self-help? The Federation, an extremely well-connected and influential group of mostly White feminists, continued to throw their energy behind efforts to keep abortion available. Still believing strongly that woman-controlled abortion was the key to liberation for all women, they returned their focus to abortion, rather than putting a great deal of emphasis on issues that groups such as the National Black Women's Health Project (NBWHP), SisterLove, and the Native American Women's Health Education Resource Center (NAWHERC) were bringing to the self-help agenda at around the same time.

When Birth Control Fails: How to Abort Ourselves Safely

After the Supreme Court legalized abortion in 1973, some self-help activists, particularly those who belonged to the Federation of Feminist Women's Health Centers, continued to practice menstrual extraction as a way to learn about and control their bodies in their own self-help groups. They typically did not practice it in woman-controlled clinics or promote it as an abortion technique. The major exception occurred in 1978, when women's health activist Barbara Ehrenreich approached the Federation to discuss the plight of a group of women in Chile who were searching for information on self-abortion after experiencing rape in prison.[4] After learning about these women, the Federation provided funding for one of its members, Suzann Gage, to publish a short, forty-eight-page book, *When Birth Control Fails: How to Abort Ourselves Safely*, which was a compilation of information on self-abortion methods. While the book included techniques ranging from the use of a bicycle pump to herbal remedies, the centerpiece was menstrual extraction. In addition to sending the information to the Chilean women, the Federation sold the book in at least fifteen countries outside of the United States. It was particularly popular in New Zealand, where the government had recently increased abortion restrictions—Gage received a "flood of requests" for it from women living there.[5]

Gage's primary goal was to create a book about self-abortion "in visual form so it could be understood by any woman, regardless of what language she spoke." Though the text was in English, in theory, women in the Chilean prison could use the detailed diagrams to perform an abortion when they needed one. Gage also wanted to "create a permanent record of self-abortion methods that have been passed down from woman to woman for centuries." In the event that other women needed to perform self-help abortions, she recalled, the Federation "wanted to preserve this information for women who had no other options."[6] The Federation pointed out in the text that it might also prove useful for women in the United States after the 1977 Hyde Amendment made it illegal to use federal funds (including Medicaid) for abortions. However, the Federation never promoted the book as a response to Hyde. They always emphasized that the Chilean women were the impetus for writing it. Although they were nominally interested in sharing information about menstrual extraction and other methods of self-abortion with women of color and poor women, their success at this time was limited.

Responses from other feminist and pro-choice groups varied. Around the United States, some woman-controlled health centers distributed copies of the book, and a number of feminist booksellers added it to their inventories.[7] On the other hand, after the Federation held a press conference to promote the book, a Planned Parenthood representative told the press that they were "in no way associated with the book."[8]

Feminist periodicals paid the most attention to the book. *off our backs* published an interview with a healthworker from a woman-controlled clinic in Europe who said that the book was "frightening!" because of its lack of attention to instrument sterilization.[9] *off our backs* reviewer Fran Moira criticized

When Birth Control Fails as dangerous and irresponsible, claiming that the abortion techniques that poor women were most likely to choose, the ones that did not require any special equipment, were the most dangerous and "described in vague and misleading terms."[10] Gage replied to the *off our backs* review, calling it a "sarcastic, distorted, sensationalized and at times, fallacious representation of self-abortion under the guise of unbiased reportage and concern for women's safety." She argued that Moira was clearly opposed to self-help and thus "sexist" in her "condescension towards any woman who has dared to abort herself."[11] Reviewers in *Healthsharing: A Canadian Women's Quarterly* wrote that they believed that there was a "pressing need for a book on self-abortion," but after reading *When Birth Control Fails* concluded that this was "*not* that book." Because of Gage's attempt to "simplify material for a wide audience," including the material on menstrual extraction, they felt that the book was too short and not detailed enough to give women adequate information about their reproductive systems.[12]

This conflict over *When Birth Control Fails* largely mirrored the debates self-help activists, especially those affiliated with the Federation, often had with the wider women's health and feminist movements. Many Federation members believed that self-help was the *key* to empowering women, and for them, self-help centered around self-exam and menstrual extraction. Other feminist and pro-choice groups believed that women did not need to know how to do abortions themselves and that it was more important to focus on keeping abortion legal and accessible. Others suggested that Federation members wanted attention and accolades. Much as the Janes had characterized Downer and Rothman as "stars" seeking admiration in the early 1970s, Moira wrote, "You are so mystified by self-importance, you cannot countenance, much less understand criticism of your book." Another *off our backs* reviewer used similar language: "Garder vos stars au frais! [Keep your stars on ice!]"[13]

Though *When Birth Control Fails* was a small-scale effort to promote menstrual extraction as an abortion technique, this incident was significant for three reasons. First, it demonstrated that the Federation was willing to promote menstrual extraction as a self-help abortion method when they believed women could not access safe and legal abortions. In spite of early 1970s attempts to couch it as a way to control their periods, when the need arose they changed their tune. Second, this incident made it clear that not all pro-choice organizations and feminist groups would respond enthusiastically to the efforts of any self-help activist who promoted menstrual extraction as an abortion method. Finally, *When Birth Control Fails* illuminates continuity within the self-help movement. The self-help movement happened largely as a response to women's lack of access to safe and legal abortions. Even as the movement expanded to address conception, contraception, menopause, HIV/AIDS, fetal alcohol syndrome, and mental health, abortion still remained a central element of women's liberation for many self-help activists, especially those affiliated with the Federation.

Once again, the Federation and many feminist clinics (for better or for worse) threw their weight behind keeping abortion available. To do this, they largely ignored other efforts to use self-help as a tool to combat women's health issues beyond abortion. As Dixon Diallo put it, abortion provision was a "heavy cross to bear," and their efforts left little room for other "crosses."

A Chill Wind Blows

The 1980s were trying years for anyone working in an abortion-providing facility. Beginning in the mid-1980s, violent incidents aimed at abortion providers in clinics and hospitals took a huge upswing.[14] During this time, a conservative backlash against the progressive advances of the 1960s and 1970s blossomed, and many members of the "New Right" organized against abortion rights. Picketers began to harass clinic and hospital clients when they were suspected of entering a facility to obtain an abortion. These women and their friends and families endured taunts, jeers, shouting, physical abuse, and other forms of harassment. Some had to deal with "sidewalk counseling," when anti-abortion activists approached women entering clinics and tried to personally persuade them not to terminate their pregnancies. In 1988, when the Democratic National Convention was held in Atlanta, thousands of men, women, and children traveled to participate in protests organized by Operation Rescue. These protests spawned others at feminist clinics around the nation, including in Yakima, Chico, Portland, Los Angeles, and Sacramento.[15]

Staff at feminist clinics devoted a great deal of time and energy to dealing with protesters and harassed clients and continuing to provide abortions in the face of this onslaught. Working with community members, they arranged escort and shuttle services to help women from their cars into the facility.[16] Many clinics became involved in long-lasting legal battles.[17] At some clinics, staff focused on chronicling the daily activities of the protesters in case these accounts were needed in court. Ultimately, twenty-two total Operation Rescue blockades in three months cost the Atlanta clinic over $100,000 to stay open, particularly because they kept having to hire new staff when workers, too stressed and fearful to continue facing these daily antagonisms, resigned. Atlanta FWHC executive director Lynne Randall said, "[Operation Rescue] drastically affected the health center, both financially and emotionally, causing a lot of stress, tension, anger, and frustration. It consumed all of our attention, energy, and money."[18] Because feminist clinics like this one felt that they must continue providing abortions at all costs, it was incredibly difficult for them to focus on other efforts. For example, Randall reported that focusing on threats while continuing to provide abortions often meant that the clinic leaders and their staff did not have time to pursue their plans to expand the provision of women's healthcare to include services such as donor insemination, and Dixon Diallo reported that efforts to combat HIV/AIDS fell by the wayside in this clinic as well.[19]

The decision to revive menstrual extraction and promote it as an early abortion procedure in the 1980s was largely a product of the clashes between anti-abortion forces and the clinics they terrorized. The "antis" pushed feminist clinics to the point that they felt they had to do something to reclaim abortion and self-help. Some feminist clinic clients linked their decision to learn menstrual extraction to the harassment they experienced at the hands of protesters. One woman told the *Atlanta Journal-Constitution* that she chose to learn the technique after Operation Rescue demonstrators "prayed for me to die, spit on me, and stepped on me."[20]

Threats to abortion rights came not only from clinic protesters but also from the Supreme Court. In 1977, the Hyde Amendment had eliminated federal funds for abortion except in cases of rape or incest, thus severely restricting low-income women's access to the procedure.[21] Over a decade later, in *Webster v. Reproductive Services*, the Court determined that the state had no obligation to provide public facilities in which abortions could be performed. In *Webster*, the Court also upheld a Missouri law requiring doctors to perform viability tests on any fetus the doctor judged to be twenty or more weeks of age, a radical departure from the precedent set by *Roe*, which mandated that the state could only regulate abortion in the second trimester to ensure the health of the mother.[22] When Justice Antonin Scalia stated that he would "reconsider and explicitly overrule *Roe v. Wade*," Justice Harry Blackmun, *Roe's* original author, wrote that "a chill wind blows" for those who support abortion rights. Calling the verdict "devastating," Downer maintained, "The ruling made it crystal clear to pro-choice supporters that women [could] no longer look to the Supreme Court to protect our most fundamental freedom, the right to choose abortion."[23]

The final impetus for feminists' embrace of menstrual extraction as an abortion technique in the late 1980s was the tightening of state laws regulating abortion. Under a controversial law in Pennsylvania, the 1989 Abortion Control Act, women considering abortion had to receive state-mandated information about abortion and state-authored information about fetal development. The act also required that a woman undergo a twenty-four-hour waiting period between consenting to an abortion and having one. Additionally, minors were required to inform at least one parent or guardian that they were having an abortion, and married women had to give prior notice to their husbands. Finally, physicians performing abortions had to turn in annual statistics reports to the state, which included the names of their patients. The Supreme Court would not test this law until 1992 in *Planned Parenthood of Southeastern Pa. v. Casey* (when they upheld most of its components), but in the late 1980s it was on the radar of many reproductive healthcare providers, who viewed it as yet another threat to abortion rights.[24] These state laws, in combination with recent Supreme Court decisions and vicious anti-abortion protests, led many self-help activists to believe that the writing on the wall said that safe and legal abortion would soon be unavailable.

No Going Back

In 1989, the Federation produced *No Going Back: A Pro-choice Perspective*, a video designed to spread the word about menstrual extraction, demonstrate self-exam, and educate women about their reproductive choices. Janet Callum of the Atlanta FWHC explained to one interested party, "With many state legislatures moving to place restrictions on abortion, there has been a resurgence of interest in this self-help technique." Although the Federation stated on several occasions that it was not meant as a how-to video, *No Going Back* contained three minutes of a live menstrual extraction. The film also included footage of a self-help group explaining the procedure.[25] Other parts of the video featured anti-abortion protesters outside of clinics. By juxtaposing footage of "antis" with footage of a menstrual extraction, the Federation made explicit the usefulness of the technique as an abortion procedure and clearly advocated menstrual extraction as a way to circumvent threats to abortion.[26] As one *Washington Post* article stated, "No step-by-step instructions are included, but anybody watching the video gathers quickly that if legal abortion were prohibited, step-by-step instructions would not be hard to come by."[27]

In reviving menstrual extraction, the Federation also sought to let the government and the American public know that an abortion technique would still be available to women if the government made medical abortions illegal. In a clear break from their pre-*Roe* rhetoric, self-help activists explicitly named menstrual extraction as an abortion procedure. One member of the Federation emphasized the film's dual purpose to the press: "It was designed to let the Supreme Court know that there are a certain number of women in society who have access to the technique of early abortion and who are going to teach other women that technique."[28]

In response to the escalating restrictions on abortion access, the Federation distributed hundreds of copies of *No Going Back*. Distributing the video proved to be a balancing act for the Federation. On one hand, they believed menstrual extraction was not a procedure to be entered into lightly. Since the early 1970s, menstrual extraction practitioners had argued that women should use this technique *only* in an advanced self-help group with other women they trusted and knew well. Self-help activists believed that to simply give women a video with instructions on how to do menstrual extraction was irresponsible. On the other hand, they also felt that it was imperative that they spread the message about menstrual extraction to as many women as possible. They advocated demonstrating the procedure in a welcoming, helpful environment with friends as the next best thing to providing safe and legal abortions in a feminist clinic setting. The group sold over 450 videos to individual women, clinics, and women's organizations and gave away a few as complimentary copies. The goal was to give presentations to accompany as many of the videos as possible.[29]

If spreading the word that the Federation was teaching menstrual extraction was as important as actually teaching it, then the Federation achieved its goal. Media coordinator Laura Brown worked to maximize the press attention the plans for the tour were receiving.[30] The Federation sent forty-six copies of *No Going Back* to the media and major news outlets including the *New York Times*, the *Washington Post*, *USA Today*, the *Los Angeles Times*, and *Newsweek*. Local papers in cities ranging from Atlanta, Cincinnati, Tampa, and St. Louis to Dallas, Salt Lake City, San Diego, Seattle, and Albany described the video, the tour, and the process of menstrual extraction and the presentations around the nation demonstrating the procedure and discussing the film. Stories about menstrual extraction also appeared on national and local television and radio. The *Dallas Morning News* noted that the motivations behind menstrual extraction were both practical and political, quoting Cynthia Pearson of the National Woman's Health Network: "Supporters want women, especially the poor, to be able to obtain abortions if the procedure becomes illegal. Menstrual extraction is intended to symbolize for state legislators—in whose hands the decision remains—how desperate the situation has become."[31]

The Federation was careful to articulate to the media that keeping abortion legal was their main goal and that they were teaching menstrual extraction as an alternative in case the option of abortion in a clinic setting became unavailable, either because a woman could not afford that option or because it became illegal. The *Los Angeles Times* quoted Downer, who said that the procedure was "a safety net, not a first choice weapon in the abortion battle." The women emphasized to the press that they were trying to prepare for doomsday. "It's the old Girl Scout's adage," Randall said to an *Atlanta Journal-Constitution* reporter. "Be prepared." She compared menstrual extraction to CPR, saying it was a skill you learn but hope you never have to use. Claiming menstrual extraction was a last resort contrasted sharply with self-help activists' earlier (1970s) stance that the procedure's primary purpose was as a technique that women could use regularly to control their periods.[32]

In 1989, Federation members began traveling to spread the word about menstrual extraction and to show *No Going Back* to audiences of women around the country.[33] For example, in April 1990, Janet Callum of the Atlanta FWHC and Deborah Fleming, the former executive director of Womancare, a woman-controlled clinic in San Diego, went on tour and facilitated five sessions across the Midwest.[34] Their first stop was the Center for Choice II, a woman-controlled clinic in Toledo, Ohio.[35] Anti-abortion terrorists had burned down the original Center for Choice clinic in 1986, and Callum and Fleming found women in Toledo keen to learn about menstrual extraction and share their stories of harassment. Carol Dunn, who hosted Callum and Fleming, told the media that the women at her clinic "felt a sense of empowerment" learning menstrual extraction, because it was a woman-controlled abortion method that was not restricted by laws or social policies.[36]

Although self-help activists maintained that menstrual extraction could help low-income women having trouble accessing a safe and legal abortion in a clinic or hospital, it was easiest to demonstrate the procedure in places where they had contacts who could cover the cost of travel and lodging and help publicize their efforts. Most Federation contacts were middle-class White feminists with a history of pro-choice activism.[37] One early 1990s article in the NBWHP's newsletter said, "The Federation has no funds for making special trips to do presentations. Travel money and accommodations must be furnished by the community that extends the invitation." The publication went on to encourage women to purchase the video for $25 if they could not afford to host Federation members in person. After Toledo, Callum and Fleming traveled to Cleveland, Ohio, where the local chapter of Refuse and Resist, a human rights activist group involved in defending abortion clinics against anti-abortion protesters, hosted them.[38] Next, they visited the Women's Studies Department at Wooster College, a small, private, Presbyterian-affiliated liberal arts school in Ohio. From there, they moved on to Chicago. Their final stop was Minneapolis, where they met with young anarchist women from the group Tornado Warning.[39]

Even though some stops on Callum and Fleming's spring 1990 tour drew much smaller numbers of people than the Federation hoped, its success lay in the media attention that it generated. For part of the tour, freelance journalist Ann Japenga traveled with Callum and Fleming. Although Japenga felt that women would be "too queasy about ME [menstrual extraction] for it to really catch on," and had "no personal burning interest in self-help," Federation members seemed to think that an in-depth media perspective on the tour was worth having, even if the journalist had a slightly "squeamish" point of view. When Japenga asked women who watched the video whether they thought they could perform a menstrual extraction if necessary, every woman reportedly answered in the affirmative.[40]

Because the legality of menstrual extraction remained somewhat dubious, by showing *No Going Back*, some self-help advocates saw themselves as engaged in acts of potential rebellion. Downer wanted pro-choice supporters to think of showing the film as a political act. She wished to "let elected officials know that if necessary, women [were] prepared to commit civil disobedience of such massive proportions that it [would] make the Prohibition era look law-abiding."[41] The purpose was to shout from the rooftops that women were arming themselves with the weapons needed to go underground if abortion became illegal. In a letter to feminist and women's health groups inviting them to purchase the video, the Federation wrote, "Won't it be great to have the Supreme Court and state legislators get the news that women are showing this film openly and defiantly in living rooms, rented halls, or at your regularly scheduled meeting?"[42]

Many of the women who learned menstrual extraction on the tour were unwilling to talk to the press about their experiences with the technique because they were unsure whether or not they were breaking the law. Those who did speak to the press often asked that they not be identified or that their names be changed, seeking to protect themselves in the face of the ambiguous legality of the procedure.[43] Some also feared that future laws could make it illegal to even share information about self-abortion. Randall told the press, "We rushed these materials out while we can still share abortion information legally."[44]

The Pro-choice Establishment Responds

Unsurprisingly, many in the pro-choice and medical communities disapproved of this revival of menstrual extraction. Groups made up largely of physicians, such as the American College of Obstetricians and Gynecologists (ACOG) and the National Abortion Federation (NAF), claimed that the procedure was dangerous and came out strongly against it.[45] A number of doctors had spoken to the press about the safety of menstrual extraction in the 1970s, but the national media attention on this do-it-yourself procedure led many more to comment in the late 1980s and early 1990s. NAF put out a statement that "menstrual extraction in advanced women's self-help groups is dangerous to the health of women."[46] It stated that menstrual extractions raised the possibility of incomplete abortions, uterine perforations, infections, sterility, and even death from accidentally rupturing an ectopic pregnancy.[47] One NAF member called menstrual extractions "unconscionable."[48] ACOG cited the same type of objections as NAF, emphasizing their stance that only a trained physician was capable of performing an abortion safely.[49]

Many self-help activists believed doctors' disapproval of the procedure stemmed more from its subversion of their authority than from concerns over safety, and the Federation tried to dismiss these concerns about menstrual extraction's safety record. "Where are the bodies?" asked Downer. "Believe me, if anyone had lost a uterus or died, it would have made headlines."[50] Rothman claimed that medical experts might be confusing menstrual extraction with other technology used by physicians, or that they were misunderstanding the way the Del-Em worked.[51] The Federation portrayed the medical community's objections to menstrual extraction as petty and territorial. A 1991 article in the *Washington Post* reported, "Proponents say doctors are reluctant to lose control over and revenues from a procedure less hazardous . . . than performing an enema."[52]

Pro-choice advocacy groups such as the National Abortion Rights Action League (NARAL) and Catholics for Free Choice (CFC) opposed promoting menstrual extraction for a different reason, emphasizing that it drew attention and resources away from the effort to keep abortion legal. "We shouldn't let the system off the hook," one CFC representative told a *Washington Post* reporter. "To say we can do abortion ourselves is to acknowledge our lack of power in the political arena."[53] These groups argued that the best way to ensure that women still had reproductive choices was to put political pressure on legislators to keep abortion legal in as many states as possible in case *Roe* were overturned.[54]

Some pro-choice groups expressed concern about menstrual extraction's appeal to low-income women who faced difficulties securing medical abortions. Especially in the wake of Hyde and *Webster*, which made it even harder for low-income women to secure abortions, they worried that women who could not afford a hospital or clinic abortion would be drawn to the procedure because it was cheap.[55] B. J. Isaacson-Jones, the director of Reproductive Health Services in the St. Louis area, argued against teaching menstrual extraction because she saw it as potentially harmful if low-income women might resort to it in desperation.[56] Others warned that rural women were more vulnerable because they were more likely to live in one of the hundreds of counties across the nation that did not have an abortion provider.[57] Members of the Federation countered that women with limited access to abortions were the very women who needed to know this method and be part of a community of self-help experts who could take care of each other if the need arose.[58] Yet there was no system in place for such women to access self-help and menstrual extraction. As women of color activists had argued for the past two decades, poor women were unlikely to take part in gynecological self-help groups or participatory groups in clinics. Though many poor women might have found menstrual extraction useful, they may not have had time, energy, access to childcare, or even transportation in order to regularly participate in a self-help group that could allow them to use menstrual extraction safely. Paradoxically, the very thing that gynecological self-help activists prized about menstrual extraction, the necessity of relying on a familiar group of other feminists to do the procedure, was an obstacle to many women who might have wanted to use it.

The NBWHP supported *No Going Back* and made its members aware of menstrual extraction.[59] Loretta Ross, then program director for the NBWHP in Atlanta, stated, "There's no denying that moving women from a medical environment to a dining room will increase risk."[60] Nonetheless, her group viewed menstrual extraction as "a safer alternative to back-alley abortions."[61] Prior to 1973, women of color died from illegal abortions at four times the rate of White women.[62] Of course, every law that threatened or restricted *Roe* was most devastating for those women who already had limited access to abortion. Ross observed that since a Del-Em could be put together for under $100, menstrual extraction was a procedure that might be accessible to women who were unable to afford other forms of abortion, giving them a possible alternative in the event that abortion became illegal or inaccessible.[63] In 1992, the NBWHP included a session on menstrual extraction at its national conference and included a full-page Q&A about *No Going Back* in a 1994 issue of its newsletter.[64] Though groups like the NBWHP wanted to extend their focus well beyond abortion, they also saw abortion as an important part of the reproductive justice agenda.

While the Planned Parenthood Federation of America did not take an official line on menstrual extraction, a few leaders expressed their opinions. As the Hyde Amendment and other restrictive legislation made abortions less accessible in the post-*Roe* era, the organization had fought a number of legislative battles to keep abortion available. In 1992, Dr. Allan Rosenfield, an obstetrician-gynecologist and former chairman of Planned Parenthood, stated that if *Roe* were overturned, the group would have to reconsider its opposition to "home abortion."[65] Yet others spoke against menstrual extraction. As a nonprofit organization, Planned Parenthood relied on federal funding and on contributions from private donors. Some donors, including the Bill and Melinda Gates Foundation, specifically earmarked their contributions so that they did not fund abortion services. Supporting a radical "home abortion" procedure would not have been in the political and financial interests of the organization.[66] Chairman of the Board of Planned Parenthood Dr. Kenneth Edelin said that while he sympathized with the cause, he viewed the use of menstrual extraction kits as "dangerous."[67]

Just as in the 1970s, local NOW chapters played an important role in disseminating information about menstrual extraction, but national spokespersons were wary. However, whereas in 1971 NOW conference organizers had forbidden Downer and Rothman to demonstrate menstrual extraction because of its ambiguous legal standing, in the late 1980s and early 1990s NOW allowed the demonstration at several annual national conferences. At the 1989 NOW conference, the Federation sold several thousand dollars' worth of materials, including the *No Going Back* video, menstrual extraction instruction manuals, and Del-Ems.[68] Although national NOW leaders refused to take an official stance on the procedure, claiming they did not want to be accused of encouraging women to do "home abortions," many NOW members and chapters took action to educate women about menstrual extraction as an early abortion procedure by inviting menstrual extraction proponents to their local meetings.[69]

The Federation relied on NOW's vast network of women to both spread the word about menstrual extraction and encourage media attention.[70] As in the 1970s, though NOW was a national organization, it had a grassroots base with local chapters that focused on issues most relevant to their communities.[71] It was no secret that local NOW chapters from Florida to Utah were meeting to discuss menstrual extraction; local papers publicized these events. One NOW representative, Janice Jochum of the Upper Pinellas County branch, maintained: "NOW has for the first time in history called for civil disobedience. We are profoundly committed to not having our rights stripped from us. But we're prepared to do what's necessary to ensure we don't go back."[72] In 1989, a NOW chapter in Dallas hosted a meeting in which over a hundred women watched *No Going Back*. At the meeting, NOW member Patricia Ireland told the press that menstrual extraction "made one thing very clear. The demand for abortions will continue and will be met one way or another."[73] At a 1992 meeting in Salt Lake City, the local NOW chapter hosted Patty Reagan, a professor of health education, to discuss menstrual extraction for the community. Reagan told audience members, "It's archaic to think we have to go back to this, but this is the '90s back-alley abortion—only . . . safer."[74] Anticipating *Planned Parenthood v. Casey*, in a press release this NOW chapter stated, "Since *Roe v. Wade* is expected to be overturned by July, this chapter meeting may well provide information that could save women's lives."[75]

In the summer of 1992, the Supreme Court announced the *Casey* verdict, ruling that the only section of the controversial 1989 Pennsylvania Abortion Control Act that was an "undue burden" was the provision that a woman had to receive consent from her husband before having an abortion. *Casey* did not overturn *Roe*, yet it rolled back many of the rights women held dear by allowing states to enforce a mandatory twenty-four-hour waiting period for an abortion, to require parental consent, to impose reporting requirements on abortion-providing facilities, and to enforce "informed consent laws," which require providers to give women scripted information about her procedure, some of which may be medically unsound. In many cases, these requirements meant that women were unable to terminate their pregnancies when they wanted to do so. Many feminists believed that *Casey* weakened *Roe* by allowing the state to have even greater involvement in abortion.[76] Because *Casey* did not entirely overturn *Roe*, the Federation scaled back its efforts to promote menstrual extraction as an abortion method over the next two years. After *Casey*, a few advocates continued to show *No Going Back* and to discuss menstrual extraction as an alternative, but widespread interest largely diminished.[77]

Although the technique itself remained largely the same, the purpose and meaning of menstrual extraction changed significantly from the 1970s to the

1990s. In the early 1970s, self-help activists claimed that menstrual extraction was simply a way for women to control their own bodies by extracting their periods whenever they wanted. Nearly two decades later, both the practical and the political reasons to learn, teach, and use menstrual extraction were different. The self-help advocates who revived menstrual extraction did so with the twin purposes of teaching women a procedure that could help them if *Roe* were overturned and demonstrating to the American public that making abortions illegal would not prevent women from ending their pregnancies. Through their efforts, many women learned the procedure, and many more learned of its existence.

"Twenty years ago, saying we were going to do our own abortions was like saying we were going to build our own nuclear bombs. Today, we know we can do it ourselves," Carol Downer said in 1992. In some ways, from the late 1960s through the early 1990s, the self-help movement came full circle. In the late 1960s and early 1970s, feminists experimented with self-help in order to make abortions available. In the twenty-year period following, women expanded the self-help movement beyond abortion to address a wide array of women's health concerns. However, for many self-help activists, woman-controlled abortion remained very important. In the decades following the revival of menstrual extraction, self-help activism continued to evolve and expand. Yet with new restrictions on abortions emerging continually, for many, the protection of abortion rights remained a critical self-help issue.

Epilogue

Self-help is a tool which works on many
levels: demystifying the medical
establishment, demystifying our bodies,
and providing the means and methods
whereby we are able to take responsibility over our health care, our environment
and our lives.
—Women's Community Health Center

The self-help movement was a political effort to revolutionize women's healthcare. Working collectively, thousands of women demystified healthcare, took
control over their bodies, and disseminated basic health information to others.
The connections between the self-help movement and current reproductive politics and healthcare debates are abundant and offer much fertile ground for
future study. Below, I offer four areas of research into such connections that
I believe warrant deeper investigation: imagined spaces created for practicing
self-help, cases in which feminist self-help efforts have been co-opted by the
medical establishment, places that have successfully adapted their use of self-
help over the past several decades, and new faces of the movement.

Imagined Spaces

Beginning in the 1990s, self-help groups increasingly took on a more "imagined"
form. That is, as activists began developing new ways of communicating with
each other, first through underground publications called "zines" and then

through the Internet, a great deal of self-help activism happened across distances, rather than in person. Literature such as pamphlets, newsletters, books, and videos had always been part of self-help activism, but whereas earlier groups typically disseminated information in print or video while simultaneously meeting in person, many 1990s and early twenty-first-century groups did not meet in person at all. Finding evidence of self-help in these places requires reconceptualizing self-help "groups."

In the 1990s, as young women across the United States began using underground publications called zines to share ideas about feminism, self-help was a popular topic.[1] In and among the crayon drawings and confrontational poetry, many zines included serious examinations of race, gender, class, and sexuality.[2] Zinesters removed themselves from the mainstream one step further than the self-help activists of the 1970s and 1980s. Eschewing respectability and credibility, they took the accessibility of health information to a new level; they were full of swear and slang. Whereas most 1970s and 1980s self-help publications prided themselves on using proper medical terminology but explained the meanings in lay-friendly language, zines often skipped this step and went directly to the lay term. For example, in an explanation of the causes of UTIs, a zine called *Doris* instructed readers, "Basically you have to make sure that anything that has touched the region around your ass . . . does not get anywhere near your vaginal region." Even if she chose to use a more technical term, the author of *Doris* usually also gave an explanation in slang terms; at the top of a list of diuretics as was the explanation "things to make you piss."[3] Similarly, *Oompa! Oompa!* explained, "In case you aren't sure, a yeast infection means your cunt itches."[4] Though the format was unique, zines carried on many of the self-help traditions that 1970s and 1980s activists had established. They shared easy-to-understand information about women's bodies and often espoused a radical critique of reproductive politics and the medical system.[5] Frequently, zine authors simply swapped their publications instead of selling them. Some zinesters created zines devoted to reviewing each other's publications and recommending them to other readers.[6] This constant back-and-forth created a shared political culture of ideas that resembled the ones created by earlier forms of feminist print culture.[7]

On the Internet, it becomes trickier to locate the politicized feminist self-help movement. Some websites express a critique of the medical system or connect their actions to feminist politics, and many online forums, message boards, and groups on social media continue the demystification and dissemination of health information. At the same time, many who access and share health information online are not engaged with feminist politics. It becomes increasingly difficult to decide where self-help continues to exist and where it has been depoliticized or co-opted. Today, anyone with access to the Internet can find information about their health. A 2013 Pew Research Center report found that a third of Americans had used the Internet to attempt to diagnose their own or a friend's condition, and 72 percent had used the Internet for general health information in the past year.[8] Though it is important to note that most of the contributors to popular websites such as WebMD are health professionals, not laypersons, most health websites are written in lay-friendly language, and any person with access to the Internet can try to self-diagnose and even self-treat.

One website that explicitly carries on the tradition of the gynecological self-help movement, especially that of the practitioners who believed that self-exam was the key to women's liberation, is the Beautiful Cervix Project. The site, run by midwife O'Nell Starkey, offers an array of gynecological self-help information, based largely around self-exam. Starkey reports between six thousand and twelve thousand views per day. Full of resources about menstruation, fertility, pregnancy, and birth, the website also includes a message board, where hundreds of women post questions for each other and for the website moderator. The centerpiece of the site is the photo gallery. There, viewers can find thousands of photos of a variety of women's cervixes throughout an entire menstrual cycle. There are also photos of cervixes taken during a Pap test, after an abortion, during pregnancy, or with conditions such as polycystic ovarian syndrome (PCOS) or cervical polyps. Starkey writes that she hopes the project will help "contradict shame and misinformation around women's reproductive health and choices." The website also sells a self-examination kit, and it ships about three to six kits a week.[9]

The array of websites that offer information about conception and donor insemination tends to be much less connected to the feminist politics of self-help. A simple Google search will unearth dozens of online groups of women who are "TTC," or "trying to conceive." These communities offer advice on the best fertility monitors and prenatal vitamins, support each other in the event of miscarriage, offer a virtual shoulder for women whose TTC journey is long and frustrating, and give advice on insemination techniques. Though these websites often do not include an explicit feminist analysis of the medical system or connect themselves directly with the self-help movement, their very existence embodies many of the ideals that 1970s and 1980s self-help activists held dear. They are a venue for women to support other women in their health and reproductive journey outside of mainstream medicine. Many suggest do-it-yourself methods of fertility awareness, including "temping" (monitoring basal body temperature to determine when ovulation has occurred), observing changes to the cervix using cervical mucus and self-exam, and using at-home ovulation predictor kits.[10] Further, thousands of women, especially lesbian women and women with transgender partners, successfully conceive at home using donor insemination techniques every year, and the Internet often connects them to potential donors and others attempting this method. Though many sperm banks require a physician's permission for women to order samples, many women circumvent this requirement by finding "known donors," either through friends or through growing websites such as Known-DonorRegistry.com. There is typically no explicit political analysis of the short-comings of the medical system in such groups, yet these women too are operating outside of mainstream medicine, and the self-help movement popularized much of the crucial information that women need in order to conduct these proce-dures at home. Though some choose the DIY way to save money, others com-ment that they pick these methods because at-home insemination is more intimate and less clinical than trying to conceive in a doctor's office, especially because their partner can be very involved in the process.[11] If demystification was a goal of the self-help movement, is the open availability of health informa-tion on the Internet one realization of that goal? Or does the existence of such information sans a political analysis or a social justice component instead repre-sent a failure of the feminist self-help movement's intentions?

Co-optation Cases

In the 1970s, some self-help practitioners claimed that *all* gynecologists should be women. In 2018, 82 percent of new U.S. ob-gyn residents were women. That number is over four times higher than it was in 1978.[12] However, even this dras-tic shift does not mean that gynecological medical care is always feminist or in line with a self-help philosophy. In hospital and clinic settings, women undoubt-edly learn about their bodies and health. However, they typically do so under the guidance of physicians and other professionals, not laywomen peers, and most do not offer a political critique of mainstream medicine.[13] Many ob-gyns and other physicians claim to offer holistic treatment options, "treating the whole woman, rather than the disease."[14] These options may include services such as massage, acupuncture, or yoga. Women's health centers that find out and address what is "on top" for women are less common. Most do not address the issues that keep so many women from even entering their doors, such as lack of health insurance, the cost of healthcare and childcare, language and cul-tural barriers, and self-esteem. The range of options in these settings would have been unimaginable without the self-help movement, but do these estab-lishments represent a complete realization of the goals of feminist self-help?[15]

Adapting Places

Many of the groups surveyed in this book have continued their work into the twenty-first century. Though some, such as the NBWHP (now the Black Women's Health Imperative) have shifted their focus to policy-oriented work, others have retained a self-help focus. Groups such as NAWHERC, for example, have found innovative ways to bring grassroots self-help efforts to local communities. Starting in 2006, KDKO, owned and operated by the Native American Community Board, on the Yankton Sioux Reservation in South Dakota, began broadcasting from the upstairs of the NAWHERC building. In addition to broadcasting GED classes and Dakota-language lessons, the station prioritizes public service announcements on health issues relevant to its listeners, including "AIDS, drug addiction, fetal alcohol syndrome, and date rape."[16] In 1992, Lillie Allen of the NBWHP created Be Present, Inc. (BPI), a multiracial organization "dedicated to building sustainable leadership for social justice."[17] Some self-help groups that were formerly part of the NBWHP became part of BPI. Members met on a regular basis to talk about "the challenges we face as individuals in a socially and politically diverse world."[18]

SisterSong Women of Color Reproductive Health Collective emerged in the late 1990s as a national coalition of indigenous women and women of color's health organizations. SisterSong pioneered the reproductive justice framework and has become the most prominent voice in shaping public discourse about health for women of color in the United States. Women from sixteen women's health organizations representing Native American, African American, Latina, and Asian and Pacific Islander women formed to concentrate on "creating a voice for grassroots women to be heard in national and international policy arenas"; among them were NBWHP, SisterLove, and NAWHERC.[19] All original member organizations agreed to use a version of psychological self-help with the rest of SisterSong. They saw it as an important way for members to work together and to avoid "act[ing] out our internalized oppressions on each other."[20]

Several of the woman-controlled clinics that organized in the 1970s still exist. A few sell self-exam kits and instructions online.[21] Progressive Health Services (PHS) in San Diego (led by Suzann Gage, Federation of Feminist Women's Health Centers member and author of several self-help books) offers "gentle, supportive and informative gynecological examinations with an emphasis on self-help and self-knowledge" and "encourage[s] your questions and active participation in your own gynecological health care."[22] Yet perhaps even more important than the remnants of an older self-help philosophy existing in these clinics are the newer responses to feminist and reproductive justice activism some of these clinics have undertaken. For example, the Atlanta FWHC acknowledges its roots as a member of the Federation and then goes on to say on its website, "Influenced by the work of reproductive justice leaders like Loretta Ross and the SisterSong Reproductive Justice Collective, we recognized the need to adopt an intersectional approach and move away from a pro-choice centered framework." Over the past several decades, this clinic has offered a multitude of services and projects developed by and for queer people, people of color, immigrants, and people from rural and low-income communities.[23]

Since the 1970s, feminists have debated what self-help means and how it should be used. Broadening the self-help agenda to interact with the reproductive justice framework necessitated redefining self-help. Is adapting to meet the needs of a community the new hallmark of self-help?

New Faces

A Los Angeles–based network of self-help researchers, the Shodhini Institute, offers self-help groups where participants do self-exam and discuss fertility consciousness.[24] Where this group differs from older self-help groups is in its celebration of and attention to transgender and gender-nonconforming bodies. This group calls itself "all-gender inclusive."[25] Shodhini members' goal is to help both cis- and transgender individuals to demystify their bodies and also to aid healthcare workers who want to learn more about the variety of bodies that exist. The Shodhini Institute explicitly claims ties to the self-help activists of the past, declaring that it is both "preserving the hard work of our predecessors . . . and tuning in to our own experience."[26] Meanwhile, some older cisgender activists continue to insist that the body is the primary marker of gender identity. For example, in 2015, Carol Downer wrote an article titled "Another Second-Wave Feminist Refuses to Be Silenced by Transgender Critics," in which she argued that trans women were not women because they "have not had the experience of being a girl or woman their whole life, so they do not have that deep bond that women have which is based on our capacity to reproduce the species; they have not been, are not presently and never will be, targets of those ruling class males who either favor or oppose population growth."[27] The conflation of womanhood with the capacity to bear children is certainly not unique to Downer. To what extent did the self-help movement and its emphasis on the body influence this mindset among a subset of feminists?

"By promoting self-help, we are preparing for the day when women will not need our services. Then, women will be their own health care providers, having control over our bodies and lives," wrote one clinic in 1976.[28] The self-help movement emerged in the 1970s because women did not have control over their own healthcare. Today, new laws and policies continue to threaten that control. Government-funded healthcare is in danger, particularly as the population of the United States continues to age. In an era when women's bodies are increasingly medicalized and when access to health and reproductive care is becoming more difficult to secure, it is more important than ever to advocate for changes in the system and to look back at women's radical attempts to control their own bodies and find alternatives to institutionalized medicine. The movement continues.

Acknowledgments

There are so many of you to whom I am forever grateful. I am in great debt to the members of my doctoral committee at the University of North Carolina, Greensboro. Lisa Levenstein encouraged me to explore a challenging reproductive rights topic and read every word of every chapter many times. During my graduate career, I left every meeting with her inspired to draw deeper connections and to probe further into the sources. Her work as a historian, a teacher, and an activist constantly inspires me. Danielle Bouchard made me think about and critique feminist thought in new ways. Her calm presence and easy-going demeanor made every interaction with her a pleasure. She has enriched this book by asking me to challenge my own assumptions about feminism. Greg O'Brien encouraged me to pursue a PhD. I am so thankful that I was able to undertake my entire graduate experience with his unwavering support and guidance. The seeds of this project began in Tom Jackson's research colloquium during my first year at UNCG. He took great interest in my research into the Jane Collective and encouraged me to look further into a reproductive health topic. He has been an invaluable ally, an inspiration, and a font of great ideas for many years.

Thank you so much to the lovely folks at Rutgers University Press and Westchester Publishing Services. I greatly appreciate Kim Guinta for taking on this project and offering loads of helpful device and Jasper Chang and Michelle Witkowski for answering endless technical questions with grace and speed. Thanks also to two anonymous reviewers for their suggestions and to Barbara Goodhouse for her eagle-eyed edits.

Dozens of archivists and reference librarians have made this experience a wonderful one. Kelly Wooten introduced me to the Atlanta Feminist Women's Health Center Records, where I first learned about the concept of self-help. She and the staff at the Sallie Bingham Center at the Rubenstein Library always made me feel welcome and excited about digging into archival sources. Kären Mason took midwestern hospitality to the next level, hosting an impromptu gathering of archivists and interns at the Iowa Women's Archives when I was visiting. Their enthusiasm for my project spurred me on through a long week of archival research. One summer, I returned home to North Carolina after a trip to Detroit, and I discovered that hundreds of the photos of archival documents that I had taken were blurry and unusable. Kristen Chinery and the staff at the Reuther Library tracked down each of these documents, then made copies and shipped them to me. Amanda Straus at Schlesinger Library on the History of Women in America and Nancy Young and Amy Hague at Sophia Smith helped me make the most of a long research trip to Massachusetts; they and their colleagues worked patiently with me as I barreled through box after box on a whirlwind self-help treasure hunt.

The research for this book would not have been possible without funding from several generous sources. I am very grateful for the Joseph Bryan Jr. Fellowship, the Sophia Smith Travel-to-Collections Fund Grant, the Linda and Richard Kerber Travel Grant for Research in the Iowa Women's Archives, the Graduate Student Research Travel Grant from the Graduate Student Association at UNCG, the Allen W. Trelease Graduate Fellowship from the History Department at UNCG, Graduate Student Travel Grants from the UNCG History Department, a Summer Research Assistantship from the UNCG Graduate School, and the Sally and Alan Cone Award from the Women's and Gender Studies Department at UNCG.

I was fortunate to attend a university that supports its graduate students wholeheartedly. "Writer's Bootcamp" organizers Laura Drew and Laura Chesak supplied a writing venue, food, support, and excellent cheerleading. Valeria Caviness tirelessly shared her formatting expertise. Mark Elliott organized an invaluable reading group; thanks so much to him and everyone in the group who read and commented on chapters. Thanks also to Mark for being the purveyor of much wisdom about the publishing process.

My colleagues have made many contributions to this project. Justina Licata has been a dear friend and a vital part of my journey as a historian. She has been wonderful company on trips to conferences, a fabulous research buddy, and an invaluable sounding board. I am immeasurably grateful for the many times she jumped at the chance to talk women's history with me. Maggy Williams Carmack has been a great long-distance colleague and friend; for months, she kept me on pace with a daily (competitive!) writing tracker, and for years, she has provided a shining example of scholarship and hard work. Joseph Ross and Ginny Summey provided boundless moral support, encouragement, and entertainment in the form of some of the sweetest kids I have ever had the privilege to know. Jamie Mize and Sarah McCartney offered advice, challenged my ideas, listened to me complain, made me laugh, and cheered me on. Classes in the UNCG History Department with Chuck Bolton, Angela Robbins, Linda Rupert, Loren Schweninger, Asa Eger, Jill Bender, Colleen Kriger, and Lisa Tolbert shaped my ability to think like a historian. The History Department at UNCG runs smoothly because of the tireless efforts of the office staff, Laurie O'Neill, Kristina Wright, and Dawn Avolio. This three-woman juggling act never ceases to amaze me. A huge thanks to the Women's and Gender Studies department at UNCG for providing new opportunities for me to grow as a feminist and scholar. Mary Morgan encouraged me to think about feminist research in new ways. Elizabeth Keathley saved me from a red-tape disaster. Sarah Hamrick and Isabell Moore kept all of us on track. Randee Goodstadt and April Birchfield at Asheville-Buncombe Technical Community College were shining examples of leadership, meticulous organization, and sheer kindness. I so appreciate their support from afar. Likewise, the encouragement from my new colleagues at Cormier Honors College at Longwood University has been exactly the right remedy for the nearing-the-finish-line blues as I have wrapped up the book. Alix Fink, Jessi Znosko, Samantha Dunn-Miller, Kevin Napier, Adam Blincoe, Alex Grabiec, and Justin Ellis—I am looking forward to many more years of working with all of you. My students here motivate and inspire me every day, and I am particularly appreciative of those in my "Bodies and Citizens" courses who gave me genuine feedback on book chapters. Thanks so much to everyone at Longwood for making me feel so welcome and happy in my new home.

None of my work would be possible without the devoted women who care for my daughter. Finding Lisa Herrick was one of my greatest strokes of luck. The wonderful staff at the Creative Learning Center and the Andy Taylor Center have continued to make me feel like an incredibly fortunate working parent.

A variety of self-help activists generously offered their time and expertise for interviews. Becky Chalker went out of her way to copy old videos and newspaper articles to share with me. In addition to spending hours answering my interview questions, she, Carol Downer, Francie Hornstein, and Yael Peskin all corresponded with me by email regularly when I had questions. Marion Banzhaf offered her home and personal papers for my research. These five women, along with Loretta Ross, Byllye Avery, Laura Jimenez, Pam Smith, and Charon Asetoyer, shared their memories and stories of the self-help movement. In addition to their time and tales, I am indebted to them for the sometimes thankless work they and dozens of other self-help activists began half a century ago in the pursuit of happier and healthier lives for women. They have enriched my life more than they will ever know.

My family made this and every struggle worthwhile; they are there in sunshine and in shadow. These folks are my hearthside. Mickey Dudley brags about me to everyone who will listen and tears up with pride at each milestone. Martha Dudley is the very definition of a strong, independent-minded woman. My sister, Julia, makes me laugh every single day and cheers me on through every hurdle. Claire Wolf, Bobby Wolf, and Zach Guca provide opportunities for debates about feminism, health, and politics. Martha and Dave Shotwell and my aunts, uncles, grandparents, and cousins support me with love and encouragement. Carter Shotwell has been my cheerleader, confidant, and favorite comedian. His commitment to feminism, social justice, and education inspires me every day, and he challenges me more than anyone else I have ever known. My daughter Caro and this book exist both in spite of and because of each other. I have already forgotten what it was like before I had the thrill of hearing her happy voice every morning, and I cannot wait to see what movements my sweetest Doodle Gal takes by storm.

Notes

Introduction

1 West Coast Sisters, "Self-Help Clinic," box 4, folder: "Self-Help Clinic (1971)," Feminist Women's Health Center Records (hereafter FWHCR), Sallie Bingham Center for Women's History and Culture, Rubenstein Rare Book & Manuscript Library, Duke University Archives, Durham, North Carolina (hereafter SBC). Dollar signs in original.

2 Beginning in the late twentieth century, some scholars and activists began categorizing feminist movements into distinct "waves," the first in the late nineteenth and early twentieth centuries, the second in the 1960s and 1970s, and the third beginning in the 1990s. According to this model, women fighting for temperance, abolition of slavery, and suffrage in the late nineteenth and early twentieth centuries constituted the first wave. Women organizing around reproductive rights, domestic violence, rape, sexual harassment, equal pay, maternity leave, sexist language, gendered divisions of labor, childcare, sexual liberation, education, pornography, prostitution, and women's health represented the second wave in the 1960s and 1970s. A conservative backlash against feminism occurred in the 1980s, and feminist activity stagnated. In the 1990s, young feminists in particular, decrying a perceived lack of diversity in the second wave, declared that they were a new, third wave. Though self-help strategies changed between the 1960s and the 1990s, the movement did not rise and fall; rather, it persisted and evolved as diverse groups of women found new ways to take control over their own bodies. This pattern fits with trends others have noticed in the feminist movement and complements studies that have problematized the "wave" metaphor. Such studies demonstrate, for example, that activism among working-class women and women of color began long before the 1960s and was not clearly distinct from earlier feminist activism. See Rosalyn Baxandall and Linda Gordon, introduction to *Dear Sisters: Dispatches from the Women's Liberation Movement*, ed. Baxandall and Gordon (New York: Basic Books, 2000); Nancy Hewitt, *No Permanent Waves: Recasting Histories of U.S. Feminism* (New Brunswick, NJ: Rutgers University Press, 2010); Kathleen A. Laughlin et al., "Is It Time to Jump Ship? Historians Rethink the Wave Metaphor," *Feminist Formations* 2:1 (2010): 76–135;

Becky Thompson, "Multiracial Feminism: Recasting the Chronology of Second Wave Feminism," *Feminist Studies* 28:2 (2002): 336–360.

3 See, for example, Jennifer Nelson, *More Than Medicine: A History of the Feminist Women's Health Movement* (New York: New York University Press, 2015); Sandra Morgen, *Into Our Own Hands: The Women's Health Movement in the United States, 1969–1990* (New Brunswick, NJ: Rutgers University Press, 2002); Sheryl Burk Ruzek, *The Women's Health Movement: Feminist Alternatives to Medical Control* (New York: Praeger, 1978); Claudia Dreifus, *Seizing Our Bodies: The Politics of Women's Health* (New York: Vintage Books, 1977); Michelle Murphy, *Seizing the Means of Reproduction: Entanglements of Feminism, Health, and Technoscience* (Durham, NC: Duke University Press, 2012); Wendy Kline, *Bodies of Knowledge: Sexuality, Reproduction, and Women's Health in the Second Wave* (Chicago: University of Chicago Press, 2010); Leslie Reagan, *When Abortion Was a Crime: Women, Medicine, and Law in the United States, 1867–1973* (Berkeley: University of California Press, 1998); Marlene Gerber Fried, *From Abortion to Reproductive Freedom: Transforming a Movement* (Boston: South End Press, 1990); Johanna Schoen, *Abortion after Roe: Abortion after Legalization* (Chapel Hill: University of North Carolina Press, 2015). See also Barbara Ehrenreich and Deirdre English, *Witches, Midwives, and Nurses: A History of Women Healers* (New York: Feminist Press at CUNY, 1973).

4 Collette Price, "The Self Help Clinic," box 2, folder 1: "Staff Meetings; Minutes, 1976–1977," Detroit Feminist Women's Health Center Records (hereafter DFWHCR), Walter P. Reuther Library Archives of Labor and Urban Affairs, Wayne State University, Detroit, Michigan (hereafter WPRL).

5 A few clinics opened before *Roe* as states began loosening their abortion restrictions, but the *Roe* verdict meant that feminists all over the United States could open woman-controlled clinics that provided abortion.

6 Because the term "self-help" has dozens of meanings, scholars from many disciplines have examined self-help in its various forms as practiced over several centuries. Some scholars have used the term "self-help" to refer to the practices involving mutual aid or reciprocal exchange of resources that human beings have devised to meet the socioeconomic needs of their communities. Others have used it to refer to the grassroots "recovery" movement of twelve-step programs such as Alcoholics Anonymous designed largely to help members deal with illnesses and addictions. Still others refer to "popular self-help," the profusion of literature and talk shows, authored and hosted largely by women that comprises entire sections of bookstores and provides much of daytime television programming. While the late twentieth-century women's health self-help movement contained elements of mutual aid, recovery, and popular self-help, its emphasis on self-help as a way to combat social inequalities and empower women in the face of pervasive sexism and racism made it unique. Other scholars of self-help in Europe and the Americas include Alfred Katz, *Self-Help in America: A Social Movement Perspective* (New York: Twayne, 1993); John Sibley Butler, *Entrepreneurship and Self-Help among Black Americans: A Reconsideration of Race and Economics* (Albany: State University of New York Press, 1991, 2005); Thomasina Jo Borkman, *Understanding Self-Help/Mutual Aid: Experiential Learning in the Commons* (New Brunswick, NJ: Rutgers University Press, 1999); Kelly Coyle and Debra Grodin, "Self-Help Books and the Construction of Reading: Readers and Reading in Textual Representation," *Text and Performance Quarterly* 13 (1993): 61–78; Maureen Ebben, "Off the Shelf Salvation: A Feminist Critique of Self-Help," *Women's Studies in*

Communication 18:2 (1995): 111–122; Debra Grodin, "The Interpreting Audience: The Therapeutics of Self-Help Book Reading," *Critical Studies in Mass Communication* 8 (1991): 404–420; Merri Lisa Johnson, *Third Wave Feminism and Television: Jane Puts It in a Box* (New York: Palgrave Macmillan, 2007); Elayne Rapping, *The Culture of Recovery: Making Sense of the Self-Help Movement in Women's Lives* (Boston: Beacon Press, 1996); Wendy Simonds, *Women and Self-Help Culture: Reading between the Lines* (New Brunswick, NJ: Rutgers University Press, 1992).

7   See Judith Walzer Leavitt, *Brought to Bed: Childbearing in America, 1750–1950* (New York: Oxford University Press, 1986); Leavitt, *Make Room for Daddy: The Journey from Waiting Room to Birthing Room* (Chapel Hill: University of North Carolina Press, 2009); Christa Craven, *Pushing for Midwives: Homebirth Mothers and the Reproductive Rights Movement* (Philadelphia: Temple University Press, 2010); Gertrude Jacinta Fraser, *African American Midwifery in the South: Dialogues of Birth, Race, and Memory* (Cambridge, MA: Harvard University Press, 1998); Holly F. Matthews, "Killing the Medical Self-Help Tradition among African Americans: The Case of Lay Midwifery in North Carolina, 1912–1983," in *African Americans in the South: Issues of Race, Class, and Gender*, ed. Hans Baer and Yvonne Jones (Athens: University of Georgia Press, 1992); Paula Michaels, *Lamaze: An International History* (Oxford: Oxford University Press, 2014); Richard W. Wertz and Dorothy C. Wertz, *Lying-In: A History of Childbirth in America* (New Haven, CT: Yale University Press, 1989).

8   See, for example, Kathy Davis, *The Making of Our Bodies, Ourselves: How Feminism Travels across Borders* (Durham: Duke University Press, 2007); Susan Wells, *Our Bodies, Ourselves, and the Work of Writing* (Stanford: Stanford University Press, 2010). Our Bodies Ourselves, "History of *Our Bodies Ourselves* and the Boston Women's Health Book Collective," accessed April 24, 2014, http://www.ourbodiesourselves.org/about/history.asp; Wendy Kline, *Bodies of Knowledge: Sexuality, Reproduction, and Women's Health in the Second Wave* (Chicago: University of Chicago Press, 2010).

9   On April 2, 2018, *OBOS* Board Chair Bonnie Shepard announced that the Boston Women's Health Book Collective would no longer publish updated print editions of the book. See "A Message About the Future of Our Bodies, Ourselves," April 2, 2018, available https://www.ourbodiesourselves.org/2018/04/a-message-about-the-future-of-our-bodies-ourselves/.

10 Stephanie Gilmore, *Groundswell: Grassroots Feminist Activism in Postwar America* (New York: Routledge, Taylor and Francis Group, 2013), 2.

11 Women's Community Health Center to Rising Sun Feminist Health Alliance, "Self-Help as an Organizing Tool," January 28, 1979, box 13, folder 9, Boston Women's Health Book Collective, Additional Records (hereafter BWHBC, Additional Records), Schlesinger Library, Radcliffe Institute, Harvard University, Cambridge, Massachusetts (hereafter Schlesinger).

12 Sharla Fett, *Working Cures: Healing, Health, and Power on Southern Slave Plantations* (Chapel Hill: University of North Carolina Press, 2002); Dorothy Roberts, *Killing the Black Body: Race, Reproduction, and the Meaning of Liberty* (New York: Pantheon Books, 1997); Loretta Ross, "African American Women and Abortion: 1800–1970," June 1, 1992, box 105, folder 13: "African American Women and Abortion: 1800–1970," National Women's Health Network Records (hereafter NWHNR), Sophia Smith Collection, Smith College, Northampton, Massachusetts (hereafter SSC).

13 Francine C. Gachupin and Jennie Rose Joe, *Health and Social Issues of Native American Women* (Santa Barbara, CA: Praeger, 2012), 57; National Institutes of Health, "Native Voices: Native People's Concepts of Health and Illness, Timeline," accessed March 31, 2015, http://www.nlm.nih.gov/nativevoices/timeline/543 .html; Barbara Gurr, *Reproductive Justice: The Politics of Health Care for Native American Women* (New Brunswick, NJ: Rutgers University Press, 2015); Andrea Smith, *Conquest: Sexual Violence and American Indian Genocide* (Cambridge, MA: South End Press, 2005); Jael Silliman et al., *Undivided Rights: Women of Color Organize for Reproductive Justice* (Cambridge, MA: South End Press, 2004); Loretta Ross and Rickie Solinger, *Reproductive Justice: An Introduction* (Oakland: University of California Press, 2017); Jennifer Nelson, *Women of Color and the Reproductive Rights Movement* (New York: New York University Press, 2003); Loretta Ross et al., *Radical Reproductive Justice: Foundation, Theory, Practice, Critique* (New York: Feminist Press at the City University of New York, 2017).

14 Andrea Tone, *Devices and Desires: A History of Contraceptives in America* (New York: Hill and Wang, 2001); Reagan, *When Abortion Was a Crime*; Laura Kaplan, *The Story of Jane: The Legendary Underground Feminist Abortion Service* (Chicago: University of Chicago Press, 1995); Adele E. Clarke, "Maverick Reproductive Scientists and the Production of Contraceptives, 1915–2000+" in *Bodies of Technology: Women's Involvement with Reproductive Medicine*, ed. Ann Rudinow Saetnan, Nelly Oudshoorn, and Marta Kirejczyk, 37–89. (Columbus: Ohio University Press, 2000); Rebecca M. Kluchin, "Pregnant? Need Help? Call Jane: Service as Radical Action in the Abortion Underground in Chicago," in *Breaking the Wave: Women, Their Organizations, and Feminism, 1945–1985*, ed. Kathleen A. Laughlin and Jaqueline L. Castledine (New York: Routledge, 2011); Melody Rose, *Safe, Legal, and Unavailable? Abortion Politics in the United States* (Washington, DC: CQ Press, 2007); Susan L. Smith, *Sick and Tired of Being Sick and Tired: Women's Health Activism in America, 1890–1950* (Philadelphia: University of Pennsylvania Press, 1995).

15 Nelson, *Women of Color and the Reproductive Rights Movement*; Silliman et al., *Undivided Rights*; Fried, *From Abortion to Reproductive Freedom*; Lynn Roberts, Loretta Ross, and M. Bahati Kuumba, "The Reproductive Health and Sexual Rights of Women of Color: Still Building a Movement," *NWSA Journal* 17:1 (2005): 93–98; Ross and Solinger, *Reproductive Justice*; Gurr, *Reproductive Justice*; Ross et al., *Radical Reproductive Justice*.

16 Ruzek, *The Women's Health Movement*; Morgen, *Into Our Own Hands*; Dreifus, *Seizing Our Bodies*; Cheryl Krasnick Warsh, *Prescribed Norms: Women and Health in Canada and the United States since 1800* (North York, ON: University of Toronto Press, 2010); Murphy, *Seizing the Means of Reproduction*; W. Kline, *Bodies of Knowledge*; Silliman et al., *Undivided Rights*; Nelson, *More Than Medicine*; Ross et al., *Radical Reproductive Justice*.

Notes to Chapter 1

Epigraph: Quoted in Maureen McDonald, "For Women Only: Alternative Health Care," *Medical Center News*, June 9, 1976, box 1, folder 40: "Correspondence, 1976," DFWHCR, WPRL.

1 Leslie Reagan, *When Abortion Was a Crime: Women, Medicine, and the Law in the United States, 1867–1973* (Berkeley: University of California Press, 1998).

2   The case was settled in their favor right after *Roe* legalized abortion. Reagan, *When Abortion Was a Crime*; Ninia Baehr, *Abortion without Apology: A Radical History for the 1990s* (Boston: South End Press, 1990).

3   Baehr, *Abortion without Apology*; Kaplan, *The Story of Jane: The Legendary Underground Feminist Abortion Service* (Chicago: University of Chicago Press, 1995); Pauline Bart, "Seizing the Means of Reproduction: An Illegal Feminist Abortion Collective—How and Why It Worked," *Qualitative Sociology* 10:4 (1987): 339–357.

4   Quoted in Bart, "Seizing the Means of Reproduction," 351–352.

5   Elaine Woo, "Creator of Device for Safer Abortions," *Los Angeles Times*, May 18, 2008, accessed February 9, 2015, http://articles.latimes.com/2008/may/18/local/me-karman18.

6   Tanfer Emin Tunc, "Designs of Devices: The Vacuum Aspirator and American Abortion Technology," *Dynamis* 28 (2008): 353–376, http://www.raco.cat/index.php/Dynamis/article/viewFile/118819/185331; Murphy, *Seizing the Means of Reproduction: Entanglements of Feminism, Health, and Technoscience* (Durham, NC: Duke University Press, 2012), 154–158.

7   Woo, "Creator of Device for Safer Abortions"; Murphy, *Seizing the Means of Reproduction*, 151. See Murphy especially for an analysis of the global bio-politics involved in menstrual regulation and Karman's use of it.

8   Tunc, "Designs of Devices," 353–376.

9   Quoted in Matthew Sobnosky, "Experience, Testimony, and the Women's Health Movement," *Women's Studies in Communication* 36 (2016): 217.

10 Francie Hornstein, interview by Hannah Dudley-Shotwell and Gill Frank, 2018.

11 Susan Brownmiller, *In Our Time: Memoir of a Revolution* (New York: Dial Press, 1999); Kathie Sarachild, "Consciousness Raising: A Radical Weapon," in *Feminist Revolution*, ed. Redstockings (New York: Random House, 1975).

12 Federation of Feminist Women's Health Centers, "Menstrual Extraction," April 13, 1978, box 6, folder: "Women's Health in Women's Hands (1 of 9)," FWHCR, SBC; Carol Downer, interview by Hannah Dudley-Shotwell, March 26, 2014.

13 Carol Downer, "No Stopping: From Pom-Poms to Saving Women's Bodies," *On the Issues Magazine*, http://www.ontheissuesmagazine.com/2011fall/2011fall_downer.php.

14 Carol Downer, interview by Hannah Dudley-Shotwell, October 27, 2015.

15 *Free to Choose: A Women's Guide to Reproductive Freedom*, (Portland, OR: Eberhardt Press, 2006).

16 "Self-Help History / Carol Downer," YouTube video, 16:41, posted by Shelby Coleman, November 6, 2014, https://www.youtube.com/watch?v=OqcGfxsLokY.

17 An IUD, or intrauterine device, is a form of long-lasting contraception that became popular in the 1970s.

18 Quoted in *Free to Choose*, 15.

19 Lorraine Rothman and Laura Punnett, "Menstrual Extraction," *Quest: A Feminist Quarterly* 4:3 (1978): 45.

20 "Menstrual Extraction" (blog), October 27, 2010, http://womenshealthinwomenshands.blogspot.com/2010/10/menstrual-extraction.html; National Women's Health Network, "Self Help Resource Guide," 1980, 23, box 50, folder 1g: "Resource Guides 1980 Self Help #7," NWHNR, SSC.

21 Downer interview, 2014; "Self-Help History / Carol Downer."

22 "Self-Help History / Carol Downer."

23 Rosetta Reitz, *Menopause: A Positive Approach* (New York: Penguin Books, 1977), 97–98.

24 "Self-Help History / Carol Downer."

25 Downer, "No Stopping."

26 McDonald, "For Women Only"; Elizabeth Fishel, "Women's Self-Help Movement: Or, Is Happiness Knowing Your Own Cervix?," *Ramparts*, November 1973, 29–32.

27 Michelle Murphy, "Immodest Witnessing: The Epistemology of Vaginal Self-Examination in the U.S. Feminist Self-Help Movement," *Feminist Studies* 30 (2004): 129.

28 Murphy, 118–130. At-home pregnancy tests did not become widely available over the counter until the late 1970s.

29 For the sake of brevity, I often refer to the group of women loosely associated with Downer who practiced gynecological self-help in the early 1970s as the West Coast Sisters. Though they occasionally published under this name, it is unclear how often they referred to themselves this way outside of print. They also sometimes referred to themselves as Self-Help One or just Self-Help Clinic.

30 Women who attended self-help groups at the Los Angeles FWHC often started their own groups in their own neighborhoods. Several other groups of women across the nation later opened other clinics using the same name, Feminist Women's Health Center. I typically distinguish these clinics from each other by using their location (e.g., Atlanta FWHC, Orange County FWHC). When the Los Angeles FWHC was founded, abortion was illegal, so the clinic focused on self-help and self-exam. See Sandra Morgen, *Into Our Own Hands: The Women's Health Movement in the United States, 1969–1990* (New Brunswick, NJ: Rutgers University Press, 2002).

31 Ancient Greeks and Romans appear to have used some form of a speculum, but the modern-day "duck-billed" version was invented by Marion Sims. See Historical Collections at the Claude Moore Health Sciences Library, University of Virginia, "Ancient Roman Surgical Instruments" exhibit, accessed November 19, 2015, http://exhibits.hsl.virginia.edu/romansurgical/.

32 Debra Brody, Sara Grusky, and Patricia Logan, "Self-Help Health," *off our backs*, July 31, 1982, 14, 17. On the history the speculum and self-help practitioners' knowledge of this history, see Gena Corea, *The Hidden Malpractice: How American Medicine Mistreats Women* (New York: Jove/HBJ, 1977); Barbara Ehrenreich and Deirdre English, *For Her Own Good: 150 Years of the Experts' Advice to Women* (Garden City, NY: Anchor Press, 1978); Margaret Sandelowski, "'The Most Dangerous Instrument': Propriety, Power, and the Vaginal Speculum," *Journal of Obstetric, Gynecological and Neonatal Nursing* 29:1 (2000): 73–82; Murphy, "Immodest Witnessing."

33 Murphy, "Immodest Witnessing," 131–132.

34 Federation of Feminist Women's Health Centers, "Menstrual Extraction."

35 West Coast Sisters, "Self-Help Clinic."

36 Marion Banzhaf, interview by Hannah Dudley-Shotwell, Skype, April 24–25, 2015; Jennifer Baumgardner, *Abortion and Life* (New York: Akashic Books, 2008). Alternate spellings include Del-um, Del'um, and Del'Em.

37 Oakland Feminist Women's Health Center, "The Proceedings of a Menstrual Extraction Conference," April 27, 1974, box 62, folder: "Participatory Clinic," FWHCR, SBC. Though the West Coast Sisters believed that a woman practicing self-exam alone in her home was better than nothing, they also felt that women would learn more by doing self-exam in a self-help group on a regular basis. See Reitz, *Menopause*, 99.

38 Lorraine Rothman, "Menstrual Extraction," 2, box 48, folder: "Menstrual Extraction," FWHCR, SBC; Murphy, "Immodest Witnessing," 118–120.

39 Feminist Women's Health Centers, "Menstrual Extraction: The Means to Responsibly Control Our Periods," n.d, box 15, folder 4: "Feminist Women's Health Center, Oakland, California," Women's Community Health Center Records (hereafter WCHCR), Schlesinger; National Women's Health Network, "Menstrual Extraction Politics," 1980, 23, box 50, folder 1g: "Resource Guides 1980 Self Help #7," NWHNR, SSC.

40 Price, "The Self Help Clinic."

41 For more on abortion activists who used arrests as a tactic to bring attention to the need for legal abortions, see Kaplan, *The Story of Jane*; Carol Joffe, "The Unending Struggle for Legal Abortion: Conversations with Jane Hodgson," *Journal of the American Medical Women's Association* 49:5 (1992): 160–164. As discussed in chapter 6, some self-help activists in the late 1980s and early 1990s flaunted menstrual extraction as an abortion procedure as a means of demonstrating that making abortion illegal did not make it disappear.

42 Laura Brown, "Blood Rumors: An Exploration of the Meaning in the Stories of a Contemporary Menstrual Practice" (PhD diss., California Institute for Integral Studies, 2002).

43 Suzann Gage, *When Birth Control Fails: How to Abort Ourselves Safely* (Hollywood, CA: Speculum Press, 1979), 17–19.

44 Because Karman was also involved in a series of population control efforts (backed by International Planned Parenthood and the United States Agency for International Development), menstrual extraction advocates believed they had additional reasons to separate themselves from Karman. See Murphy, *Seizing the Means of Reproduction*.

45 "Feminist Women's Health Centers," February 1973, box 2, folder 25: "FWHC Early Political Papers 1976," DFWHCR, WPRL; West Coast Sisters, "Self-Help Clinic."

46 Quoted in Brown, "Blood Rumors," 196.

47 Lorraine Rothman, "Menstrual Extraction," in National Women's Health Network Resource Guide 7, *Self-Help*, box 50, folder 1g: "Resource Guides 1980 Self Help #7," NWHNR, SSC.

48 Feminist Women's Health Centers, "Menstrual Extraction."

49 Brown, "Blood Rumors," 15.

50 Christine Eubank, "The Speculum and the Cul-de-Sac: Suburban Feminism in the 1960s and 1970s, Orange County, California" (PhD diss., University of California, Irvine, 2013), 106–107.

51 Downer, "No Stopping."

52 Stephanie Gilmore, *Groundswell: Grassroots Feminist Activism in Postwar America* (New York: Routledge, Taylor and Francis Group, 2013).

53 Rothman, "Menstrual Extraction," FWHCR, SBC.

54 Eberhardt Press, "Free to Choose," 18.

55 Carol Downer and Rebecca Chalker, *A Woman's Book of Choices: Abortion, Menstrual Extraction, RU-486* (New York: Seven Stories Press, 1992), 117.

56 Self Help Clinic One, "Self-Help Clinic Paramedic Politics," box 2, Health Collection, SSC.

57 Dido Hasper, interview by Gayle Kimball, 1981, http://www
.womenshealthspecialists.org/images/pdf/interview%20with%20dido%20hasper
.pdf; Delia M. Rios, "Abortions at Home: Women Fearing End of *Roe vs. Wade*
Learn Procedure, Part 1 of 2," *Dallas Morning News*, August 4, 1991, 1A.

58 Rios, "Abortions at Home"; Morgen, *Into Our Own Hands*, 7–8. Self-help activists continued to rely on NOW in the next several decades as a source of staff and clients for woman-controlled clinics. Ties with NOW would again prove important in the late 1980s and early 1990s when self-help activists revived menstrual extraction.

59 Gena Corea, "Self-Help Groups," in National Women's Health Network Resource Guide 7, *Self-Help*, box 50, folder 1g: "Resource Guides 1980 Self Help #7," NWHNR, SSC.

60 That said, from its inception, NOW was interested in a range of social justice issues facing women, including poverty and racial inequality. Histories of the organization that have focused primarily on its national spokeswomen have sometimes obscured these efforts. See Gilmore, *Groundswell*.

61 Murphy, "Immodest Witnessing"; Silliman et al., *Undivided Rights: Women of Color Organize for Reproductive Justice* (Cambridge, MA: South End Press, 2004); Nelson, *Women of Color and the Reproductive Rights Movement* (New York: New York University Press, 2003); Johanna Schoen, *Choice and Coercion: Birth Control, Sterilization, and Abortion in Public Health and Welfare* (Chapel Hill: University of North Carolina Press, 2005); L. Ross et al., *Radical Reproductive Justice: An Introduction* (Oakland: University of California Press, 2017); Gurr, *Reproductive Justice: The Politics of Health Care for Native American Women* (New Brunswick, NJ: Rutgers University Press, 2015).

62 Judith Aliza Hyman Rosenbaum, "Whose Bodies? Whose Selves? A History of American Women's Health Activism, 1968–Present" (PhD diss., Brown University, 2004), 120.

63 Anne M. Valk, *Radical Sisters: Second-Wave Feminism and Black Liberation in Washington, D.C.* (Urbana: University of Illinois Press, 2008).

64 Quoted in Rosenbaum, "Whose Bodies? Whose Selves?"

65 Cindy Pearson, Cecile Latham, and Kris Shepos-Salvatore, "Menstrual Extraction: Women Take Control," *off our backs*, April 1992, 1–3, 23.

66 Quoted in Eubank, "The Speculum and the Cul-de-Sac," 111.

67 Lolly Hirsch, *The Witch's Os* (Stamford, CT: New Moon Publications, 1972), 22.

68 Mailer, a prolific author, was well known for his views against women's liberation. Elizabeth Campbell, "Why Self Health," *Women's Health Care: Nursing Dimensions* 7:1 (1975): 68–69, Women's Newsletter and Periodical Collection (hereafter WNPC), Schlesinger.

69 The clinic went by various names including the Los Angeles Feminist Women's Health Center, the Feminist Women's Health Center, and the Self-Help Clinic.

70 West Coast Sisters, "Women's Self Help Clinic: Or What to Do While the Physician Is on His Bread-Filled Ass," 1971, box 62, folder: "Participatory Clinic," FWHCR, SBC.

71 "Police Raid Women's Do It Yourself Clinics," *Los Angeles Sentinel*, September 28, 1972, A1.

72 Hasper interview, 1981. Some sources report that two women attending the group were undercover policewomen. See New Moon Publications, "SOS SOS SOS, Save Our Sisters!," *Monthly Extract: An Irregular Periodical* 1:1-a (September 1972), WNPC, Schlesinger.

73 "Police Raid Women's Do It Yourself Clinics," A1.

74 Stephanie Caruana, "Great Yogurt Conspiracy," *off our backs*, January 1973, 7.

75 Feminist Women's Health Center, "Feminist Rape," September 23, 1972, box 3, Health Collection, SSC.

76 New Moon Publications, "SOS SOS SOS, Save Our Sisters!"

77 Corea, "Self-Help Groups."

78 Sheryl Kendra Ruzek, "The Women's Health Movement: Finding Alternatives to Traditional Medical Professionalism" (PhD diss., University of California, Davis, 1977), 103–104.

79 Eubank, "The Speculum and the Cul-de-Sac," 129.

80 "Practicing Health without a License," November 16, 1978, box 6, folder: "Women's Health in Women's Hands (7 of 9)," FWHCR, SBC.

81 Corea, "Self-Help Groups."

82 Federation of Feminist Women's Health Centers, "The Grassroots of Self-Help," box 3, folder: "Lesbian/Women's Health Organizations," Lesbian Health Resource Center (hereafter LHRC), SBC. Emphasis in original.

83 Quoted in Reitz, *Menopause*, 98.

84 Judith A. Houck, "The Best Prescription for Women's Health: Feminist Approaches to Well-Woman Care," in *Prescribed: Writing, Filling, Using, and Abusing the Prescription in Modern America*, ed. Jeremy Greene and Elizabeth Siegel Watkins (Baltimore: Johns Hopkins University Press, 2012), 134–135.

85 "Police Raid Women's Do It Yourself Clinics," A1.

86 Ruzek, "The Women's Health Movement," 105.

87 Caruana, "Great Yogurt Conspiracy." Other sources spell Dalton's first name "Sharyn." See Mariana Hernandez, "Self-Help Clinic Director Acquitted in L.A.," *The Militant*, December 22, 1972, box 2, Health Collection, SSC.

88 Quoted in Corea, "Self-Help Groups."

89 "Verdict Believed Near in Coast Trial of Feminist Charged with Practice of Medicine without License," *New York Times*, December 3, 1972.

90 New Moon Publications, "SOS SOS SOS, Save Our Sisters!"

91 Hasper interview, 1981, 15; Reitz, *Menopause*, 98; Morgen, *Into Our Own Hands*, 23–26.

92 Quoted in Eubank, "The Speculum and the Cul-de-Sac," 112.

93 The AMA (American Medical Association) is the largest association of physicians in the United States. The ACOG (American College of Obstetricians and Gynecologists) is a professional association of ob-gyns. Brody, Grusky, and Logan, "Self-Help Health," 14, 17.

94 Reproductive Rights National Network, "Rough Road Ahead," *off our backs*, August-September 1981, 10, 17.

95 Ellen Frankfort, *Vaginal Politics* (New York: Quadrangle Books, 1972), xiii–xiv.

96 Eubank, "The Speculum and the Cul-de-Sac," 111.

97 Susan Bartlett, "Why Gynecological Self-Help," *WomenWise*, Fall 1978, 2, box 6, Health Collection, SSC.

98 Price, "The Self Help Clinic."

99 Avery later helped develop a version of self-help that women of color used to deal with internalized racism and sexism. See chapter 5.

100 Avery was so struck by the need for women to find "harmony" with their periods that she later created a film, *On Becoming a Woman: Mothers and Daughters Talking Together*, to show women and girls dialoguing honestly about menstruation. Avery refers to menstrual extraction as "aspiration," highlighting the confusion over the term even within the women's health movement. The other two women who founded the Gainesville Women's Health Center were Judith Levy and Margaret Parrish. Byllye Avery, interview by Loretta Ross, Voices of Feminism Oral History Project, Sophia Smith Collection, Smith College, 2005.

101 Frankfort, *Vaginal Politics*, xii. Interestingly, Frankfort acknowledged in her book (226) that the majority of the letters she received from physicians after writing a piece on menstrual extraction were about their fears at women holding such autonomy over their bodies, not about the actual physical dangers of the procedure.

102 Frankfort, xvi.

103 Dorothy Tennov, "A Review by Dorothy Tennov of Ellen Frankfort's Book: *Vaginal Politics*," *Feminist Women's Health Center Report* 1:3 (1977): 13, box 2, folder 4: "FWHC Annual Report 1974–78," DFWHCR, WPRL.

104 Kaplan uses pseudonyms (Pat and Monica) for the West Coast Sisters who visited the Jane Collective. See Kaplan, *The Story of Jane*, 197–202.

105 Kaplan, 197–202.

106 Kaplan, 197–202.

107 Downer interview, 2014.

108 West Coast Sister, "Self-Help Clinic, Part II," Feminist Women's Health Centers, 1971, quoted in Ruzek, "The Women's Health Movement," 101–102.

109 *NOW Newsletter* 2:12 (December 1971), quoted in Eubank, "The Speculum and the Cul-de-Sac," 115; capitalization in original.

110 Philadelphia Women's Health Collective, "The Philadelphia Story: Another Experiment on Women," box 14, folder 8, "Feminist Women's Health Center, Los Angeles, 1974–1977; includes correspondence with and reports by Carol Downer," WCHCR, Schlesinger.

111 Woo, "Creator of Device for Safer Abortions."

112 "Controversies in Birth Control," July 19, 1978, box 6, folder: "Women's Health in Women's Hands (2 of 9)," FWHCR, SBC.

113 Murphy, *Seizing the Means of Reproduction*.

114 "Controversies in Birth Control," FWHCR, SBC.

115 Federation of Feminist Women's Health Centers, "Menstrual Extraction"; "Synopsis: The Activities of Harvey Karman," *Feminist Women's Health Center Report*, 8, box 4, Health Collection, SSC; Eubank, "The Speculum and the Cul-de-Sac," 115.

116 "Synopsis," *Feminist Women's Health Center Report*; Ruzek, "The Women's Health Movement." Downer also later recounted to me that she knew Peggy Grau, a woman who worked as a receptionist in Karman's clinic. Downer believed that Grau had never shown any interest in menstrual extraction or abortion at all, and that Karman was writing under her name. See Downer interview, 2015.

117 "Synopsis," *Feminist Women's Health Center Report*; Helen Koblin, "Vaginal Politics: Harvey Karman, Abortionist," *Los Angeles Free Press*, June 9, 1972, box 8, Health Collection, SSC.

118 "Synopsis," *Feminist Women's Health Center Report*.

119 She originally filed for the patent in 1971, but it took several years to finalize.

120 Tunc, "Designs of Devices," 353–376; "Notes on Meeting with Attorney," August 25, 1989, box 62, folder: "ME Coverage (2 of 4)," FWHCR, SBC; Tacie Dejanikus, "Menstrual Extraction," *off our backs*, December 1972, 4–5; United States Patent 3,828,781, August 13, 1974; West Coast Sisters, "Self-Help Clinic."

121 Judith Bourne et al., "Medical Complications from Induced Abortion by the Super Coil Method," *Health Services Reports* 89:1 (May-June 1974), https://www.ncbi.nlm.nih.gov/pmc/articles/PMC1616242.

122 Abortion law in Pennsylvania was in flux at this point, and some doctors were openly offering abortions in clinics. See Kaplan, *The Story of Jane*, 239. Gosnell too became a controversial figure in the abortion rights movement. In 2010, the FBI and Pennsylvania Department of Health raided and shut down his clinic over suspicions of illegal drug activity. When the officials discovered that the clinic did not comply with state and federal laws, Gosnell went to trial. He was convicted of three counts of murder of babies born alive in the clinic. Pro-choice activists used this case to push for better access to abortions so that women did not have to resort to providers like Gosnell. Pro-life activists used this case as a call for stronger clinic regulations. Sarah Kliff, "Kermit Gosnell," *Washington Post*, April 15, 2013; Jon Hurdle and Trip Gabriel, "Philadelphia Abortion Doctor Guilty of Murder in Late-Term Procedures," *New York Times*, May 13, 2013.

123 Kaplan, *The Story of Jane*, 197–202.

124 Tacie Dejanikus, "Super-coil Controversy," *off our backs*, May 1973, 2–3, 11.

125 Others called the event the Mother's Day Massacre, because it happened on May 14, Mother's Day. Kaplan, *The Story of Jane*, 241; Philadelphia Women's Health Collective, "The Philadelphia Story."

126 Downer denied that her group had any connection to "The Philadelphia Story." Downer interview, 2015.

127 Kaplan, *The Story of Jane*, 242. It is unclear whether the Janes believed the West Coast Sisters wrote the paper and published it under the name of the Philadelphia Women's Health Collective or whether they thought the West Coast Sisters just encouraged it.

128 Kaplan, 197–202; Philadelphia Women's Health Collective, "The Philadelphia Story."

129 Philadelphia Women's Health Collective, "The Philadelphia Story."

130 Ultimately, Karman was charged with eleven counts of performing illegal abortions and eleven counts of practicing medicine without a license. He was convicted of two counts and fined $500. Philadelphia Women's Health Collective, "The Philadelphia Story."

131 Kaplan, *The Story of Jane*, 241.

132 McDonald, "For Women Only."

Notes to Chapter 2

Epigraph: Banzhaf interview, 2015.

1 Banzhaf interview.

2 Though abortion providers all over the country faced similar staff-related struggles, in woman-controlled clinics, "burnout" and interstaff conflict were often intensified by these clinics' attempts at egalitarianism.

3 Reagan, *When Abortion Was a Crime.*

4 This group included many, but not all, of the West Coast Sisters, as well as several other California women who had begun to practice self-help. See Nelson, *More Than Medicine*, on neighborhood clinics.

5 Francie Hornstein, "Lesbian Healthcare," in *Lesbian Health Activism: The First Wave; Feminist Writings from the Early Lesbian Health Movement*, December 1973, Feminist Health Press, box 9, folder 28: "Brochures/Factsheets/ Publications: Publication: *Lesbian Health Activism: The First Wave*, 2001," Records of the Mautner Project, Schlesinger.

6 Eubank, "The Speculum and the Cul-de-Sac," 106; Self Help Clinic One, "The Brown Baggers of the NOW Convention"; Nelson, *More Than Medicine.*

7 Some women were able to open clinics before either of these cases was decided, because they lived in states that liberalized abortion laws before 1973 or because they offered only gynecological services, not abortion. Among these clinics were the Los Angeles FWHC, the Somerville Women's Health Center (in Massachusetts), the Emma Goldman Clinic in Chicago (not to be confused with the EGC in Iowa City, which opened in 1974), and the Elizabeth Blackwell Women's Health Center in Minneapolis.

8 Katarina Keane, "Second-Wave Feminism in the American South, 1965–1980" (PhD diss., University of Maryland, College Park, 2009), 177–178.

9 I refer to the clinics operating with a "self-help philosophy" interchangeably as "woman-controlled clinics," "feminist clinics," and "feminist health centers." The staff at these clinics referred to them in all of these ways.

10 Morgen, *Into Our Own Hands*; Ruzek, *The Women's Health Movement.*

11 Anne Enke, *Finding the Movement: Sexuality, Contested Space, and Women's Activism* (Durham, NC: Duke University Press, 2007); Kristen Hogan, *The Feminist Bookstore Movement: Lesbian Antiracism and Accountability* (Durham, NC: Duke University Press, 2016).

12 Among these new clinic leaders were Lorraine Rothman and Laura Brown, the daughter of Carol Downer. Some women, such as Francie Hornstein, even moved to California after seeing a self-help presentation so that they could join the FWHCs there. Francie Hornstein, interview by Hannah Dudley-Shotwell, June 2, 2015.

13 Timeline of Women's Community Health Center, box 1, folder: "Women's Community Health Center, History, Bylaws, and Newsletters, 1975–1976 and undated," Carol Hodne Records (hereafter Hodne Records), Iowa Women's Archives, University of Iowa Archives, University of Iowa Libraries, Iowa City, Iowa (hereafter IWA).

14 Eubank, "The Speculum and the Cul-de-Sac," 124–125.

15 "Minutes," June 4, 1974, box 13, folder: "General Minutes, January 1973–Sept. 1974," Emma Goldman Clinic for Women (Iowa City) Records (hereafter EGCR), IWA.

16 "In the Beginning . . . A Herstory of the Women's Community Health Center," box 1, folder 13: "Annual Reports, 1975–1977, 1979," WCHCR, Schlesinger.

17 Marlene Perrin, "Nye Celebrates I. C. Clinic Milestone," *The Gazette* (Cedar Rapids/Iowa City), August 3, 2003, J1.

18 Participatory groups went by a variety of names in different clinics. "Orientation/ Training Manual for Clinic Employees," April, 1984, box 10, folder: "Orientation/Training Manual for Clinic Employees," FWHCR, SBC.

19 Many clinics used the term "healthworker" to refer to the laywomen who did the bulk of the work in clinics. Some used "paramedics," or simply "clinic staff."

20 "Orientation/Training Manual for Clinic Employees."

21 West Coast Sisters, "Self-Help Clinic."

22 Kathleen I. MacPherson, "Feminist Praxis in the Making: The Menopause Collective" (PhD diss., Brandeis University, 1986), 226.

23 "Orientation/Training Manual for Clinic Employees."

24 Brody, Grusky, and Logan, "Self-Help Health," 14.

25 Marion Banzhaf, interview by Sarah Schulman, April 18, 2007, ACT UP Oral History Project, accessed August 6, 2019, http://www.actuporalhistory.org/interviews/images/banzhaf.pdf.

26 Sheryl K. Ruzek, "Emergent Modes of Utilization: Gynecological Self-Help," in *Women's Health Care*, ed. Karren Kowalski, WNPC, Schlesinger.

27 Laws varied by state, so some clinics were also able to employ nurse practitioners and physician's assistants to write prescriptions.

28 See Carole E. Joffe, *Dispatches from the Abortion Wars: The Costs of Fanaticism to Doctors, Patients, and the Rest of Us* (Boston: Beacon Press, 2009); Carole E. Joffe, *Doctors of Conscience: The Struggle to Provide Abortion before and after Roe v. Wade* (Boston: Beacon Press, 1995).

29 McDonald, "For Women Only."

30 Federation of Feminist Women's Health Centers, "The Drape and Stirrups," box 62, folder: "Participatory Clinic," FWHCR, SBC.

31 Frankfort, *Vaginal Politics*, xii.

32 "Federation of Feminist Women's Health Centers: The Participatory Clinic," box 62, folder: "ACOG Action," FWHCR, SBC.

33 Feminist Women's Health Center, "A Visit to a Clinic or Physician," August 15, 1978, box 6, folder: "Women's Health in Women's Hands (8 of 9)," FWHCR, SBC.

34 Daphne Spain, *Constructive Feminism: Women's Spaces and Women's Rights in the American City* (Ithaca, NY: Cornell University Press, 2016), 123. Also see Spain for a thorough account of clinics as feminist spaces.

35 Planned Parenthood "Cervical Cap (FemCap)," accessed March 11, 2014, http://www.plannedparenthood.org/health-topics/birth-control/cervical-cap-20487.htm; "Specific Duties of Nurse in Abortion Clinic," box 9, folder: "Specific Duties of Nurse in Abortion Clinic," 5, FWHCR, SBC.

36 Banzhaf interview, 2015. The home pregnancy test became available in the United States in 1976. Office of NIH History, "A Timeline of Pregnancy Testing," accessed December 17, 2015, https://history.nih.gov/exhibits/thinblueline/timeline.html.

37 "Shortened Abortion Group #1," box 4, folder: "Shortened Ab Group," FWHCR, SBC.

38 "Services of the Feminist Women's Health Center . . . Woman's Choice Clinic," 1976, box 1, folder 40: "Correspondence, 1976," DFWHCR, WPRL.

39 Banzhaf interview, 2015; "Service Protocols," April 1987, box 7, folder: "Protocols—Old," FWHCR, SBC; Feminist Women's Health Center Review, "Feminists Wanted," December 1979, box 15, folder 6: "Feminist Women's Health Center, Santa Ana, Calif., 1974–1979," WCHCR, Schlesinger.

40 "Service Protocols"; "Feminist Women's Health Center Clinic Guidelines / Standardized Procedures," April 1984, box 10, folder: "Clinic Guidelines / Standardized Procedures," FWHCR, SBC.

41 "Service Protocols."
42 "Feminist Women's Health Center Healthworking in the Exam Room / First Trimester Abortion Procedures Training," October 1998, box 8, folder: "First Trimester Explanation / Authorization & Consent," FWHCR, SBC.
43 "Service Protocols."
44 See Wendy Simonds, *Abortion at Work: Ideology and Practice in a Feminist Clinic* (New Brunswick, NJ: Rutgers University Press, 1996), for more on the daily struggles of working in a feminist abortion clinic.
45 Feminist Women's Health Center Review, "Feminists Wanted."
46 Sandra Morgen and Alice Julier, "Women's Health Movement Organizations: Two Decades of Struggle and Change," June 27, 1991, box 1, folder 9: "Articles, 1979–99," NWHNR, SSC, 9.
47 Beverly Smith, "Development of an Ongoing Data System at a Women's Health Center," 1976, box 1, folders 1.4 and 1.5: "Development of an Ongoing Data System," WCHCR, Schlesinger, 107.
48 Morgan and Julier, "Women's Health Movement Organizations," 9; Women's Community Health Center, "A Report from Women's Community Health Center," *Quest: A Feminist Quarterly* 4:1 (Summer 1977): 14, box 13, folder 2: "Federation of Feminist Women's Health Centers, 1972–1980," WCHCR, Schlesinger.
49 As many as twenty woman-controlled clinics joined the Federation over the next decade. Women's Health Specialists: The Feminist Women's Health Centers of California, accessed April 4, 2014, http://www.womenshealthspecialists.org/.
50 Hasper interview, 1981.
51 The group of clinics discussed here did not formally become "the Federation" until a year after this incident, though they were allied closely together long before that. For simplicity's sake, I refer to them here as "Federation clinics." See Morgen, *Into Our Own Hands*, 24–25.
52 "What Is 'Feminist' Health?," *off our backs*, June 1974, 2–5.
53 Sharon Johnson to All Institute Participants, "The Relationship between the FWHC and the Institute Program," July 1, 1974, box 14, folders 8–10: "Feminist Women's Health Center, Los Angeles, 1974–1977; includes correspondence with and reports by Carol Downer," WCHCR, Schlesinger.
54 "What Is 'Feminist' Health?," 2–5; Eubank, "The Speculum and the Cul-de-Sac," 121.
55 "What Is 'Feminist' Health?," 2–5.
56 Francie Hornstein to Jennifer, Courtney, Lolly, Mary, Ellen, Linda, and all, June 10, 1974, box 14, folders 8–10: "Feminist Women's Health Center, Los Angeles, 1974–1977; includes correspondence with and reports by Carol Downer," WCHCR, Schlesinger.
57 "What Is 'Feminist' Health?," 2–5.
58 "What Is 'Feminist' Health?," 2–5.
59 Carol Downer, "What Makes the Feminist Women's Health Center 'Feminist,'?," *off our backs* 4:7 (June 1974): 4.
60 "What Is 'Feminist' Health?," 2–5. Emphasis in original.
61 "What Is 'Feminist' Health?," 2–5.
62 Miriam Frank, Carole Kellogg, Cathy LaDuke, Kaye Otter, Connie Cronin, Nikki Muller, Mary Jo, Denise Jacques, and Gracia Holt, "More FWHC," *off our backs* 4:9 (August-September 1974): 22.

63 Francie Hornstein to "Folks," June 10, 1974, box 14, folders 8–10: "Feminist Women's Health Center, Los Angeles, 1974–1977; includes correspondence with and reports by Carol Downer," WCHCR, Schlesinger.

64 Carol Downer, Lorraine Rothman, and Eleanor Snow, "FWHC Response," *off our backs*, August-September 1974, 17–20.

65 "Positions of Greatness," *off our backs*, June 30, 1974, 1.

66 Frank et al., "More FWHC," 22; Dell Williams, Jane Field, Teresa Hoover, Joanne Parrent, Valerie Klaetke, Deborah A. Davis, Cathy Cade, and Brenda Carter, "Responses to FWHC," *off our backs*, July 1974, 26.

67 Williams et al., "Reponses to FWHC," 26.

68 Quoted in Rosenbaum, "Whose Bodies? Whose Selves?," 68.

69 See Terry Mizrahi, "Women's Ways of Organizing: Strengths and Struggles of Women Activists over Time," *Affilia: Journal of Women and Social Work* 22:1 (2007): 39–55; Janice Ristock, "Feminist collectives: The Struggles and Contradictions in Our Quest for a 'Uniquely Feminist Structure," in *Women and Social Change: Feminist Activism in Canada*, ed. Jeri Wine and Janice Ristock (Halifax: James Lorimer and Company, 1991), 41–55; Margaret Strobel, "Organizational Learning in the Chicago Women's Liberation Union," in *Feminist Organizations: Harvest of the New Women's Movement*, ed. Myra Ferree and Patricia Martin (Philadelphia: Temple University Press, 1995), 145–164; Kathleen Iannello, *Decisions without Hierarchy: Feminist Interventions in Organization Theory and Practice* (New York: Routledge, 1992); Jo Freeman, "The Tyranny of Structurelessness," in *Dear Sisters: Dispatches from the Women's Liberation Movement*, ed. Rosalyn Baxandall and Linda Gordon (New York: Basic Books, 2000), 73–75.

70 Quoted in Ruzek, "The Women's Health Movement," 137.

71 Political Beliefs of the Feminist Women's Health Center, box 62, folder: "Participatory Clinic," FWHCR, SBC.

72 Yet debates about what constituted "feminist" self-help did not end with questions about leadership. In 1979, a Cape Cod women's group called Abortion Rights Movement—Women's Advocacy Service (ARM-WAS), which counseled and provided patient advocates for local women seeking abortions in Boston, approached the Women's Community Health Center (WCHC) to form a partnership to bring women to WCHC. The two groups disagreed over whether patient advocates were necessary in feminist, self-help-oriented settings. WCHC employees argued that advocates were not needed and that providing them would even *disempower* women from advocating for themselves. "It . . . implies a lack of trust for our work to want to advocate in a woman-controlled self-help setting. We define feminist self-help as encouraging women to take more power and control in our lives, facilitating a mutual sharing and validation of our experiences, and challenging the assumptions and power structure that have attempted to keep us from doing these things. In view of this, we do not encourage women to become reliant on any one particular healthworker for support or information. . . . We also hope to see women who come here supporting each other and advocating for themselves." ARM-WAS disagreed, arguing that the WCHC was too rigid and not living up to feminist principles: "We must address your philosophy that advocacy is not necessary in your clinic. We believe that in any clinic, feminist self-help or not, so long as physicians do the abortions and medical procedures and the state regulates how we run our clinics, outside advocates should be encouraged." Quoted in Rosenbaum, "Whose Bodies? Whose Selves?," 68.

73 Benita Roth, *Separate Roads to Feminism: Black, Chicana, and White Feminist Movements in America's Second Wave* (New York: Cambridge University Press, 2004).

74 Enke, *Finding the Movement*; Valk, *Radical Sisters*.

75 Enke, *Finding the Movement*.

76 Roughly $350 at the time of this publication. This works out to about $18,000 a year.

77 Women's Community Health Center, "A Report from Women's Community Health Center," 20.

78 "Feminist HealthCare: A Continuum," *Santa Cruz Women's Health Center Newsletter*, no. 39 (Fall 1985), carton 7, WNPC, Schlesinger.

79 Celine, "A View on Feminist Clinics," *off our backs*, August 31, 1976, 22–23; Banzhaf interview, 2015.

80 Avery interview, 2005.

81 Avery interview; Keane, "Second-Wave Feminism in the American South," 201.

82 Banzhaf interview, 2015.

83 Hornstein interview, 2018.

84 Women's Community Health Center, "Self-Help as an Organizing Tool."

85 Pam Smith, interview by Hannah Dudley-Shotwell, July 26, 2017. Interestingly, when I corresponded with Byllye Avery via email in July 2017 about this incident, she had no memory of it. As she pointed out, "That was a long time ago for all of us." I relate Smith's memory of the event here, even though the details are scant, because it is in line with similar conflicts over gynecological self-help and race at other clinics.

86 Banzhaf interview, 2015; Teresa Barnes, "Not until Zimbabwe Is Free Can We Stop to Think about It: The Zimbabwe African National Union and Radical Women's Health Activists in the United States, 1979," *Radical History Review*, no.119 (2014): 53–71.

87 "Gyn Committee Meeting," November 28, 1974, box 13, folder: "Clinic Committee, 1974–1977," EGCR, IWA; "Gyn Committee Meeting," December 6, 1974, box 13, folder: "Clinic Committee, 1974–1977," EGCR, IWA.

88 Banzhaf interview, 2007, 21–22.

89 Hornstein interview, 2015. Emphasis in inflection.

90 Pam Smith, interview by Sinister Wisdom, http://www.sinisterwisdom.org /SW93Supplement/Smith. Smith later related to me via email in March 2019 that this was a bit of an exaggeration, and *most* of the women came out as lesbians, whereas a few stayed in heterosexual relationships.

91 Paula Klein, "Health Needs Assessment in a Lesbian Community," September 10, 1980, box 44, folder: "Lesbian Health Issues," EGCR, IWA.

92 Hornstein, "Lesbian Healthcare."

93 Berkeley Women's Health Collective, "Lesbian Clinic" flyer in *Lesbian Health Activism: The First Wave; Feminist Writings from the Early Lesbian Health Movement*, December 1973, Feminist Health Press, box 9, folder 28: "Brochures/Factsheets/ Publications: Publication: *Lesbian Health Activism: The First Wave*, 2001," Records of the Mautner Project, Schlesinger; Feminist Women's Health Center, "Lesbian Well-Woman Clinic," flyer in *Lesbian Health Activism: The First Wave; Feminist Writings from the Early Lesbian Health Movement*, December 1973, Feminist Health Press, box 9, folder 28: "Brochures/Factsheets/Publications: Publication: *Lesbian Health Activism: The First Wave*, 2001," Records of the Mautner Project, Schlesinger.

94 Gay Women's Liberation Collective, "In Amerika They Call Us Dykes," quoted in "Lesbian Health Care: Issues and Literature," in *Lesbian Health Activism: The First Wave; Feminist Writings from the Early Lesbian Health Movement,* December 1973, Feminist Health Press, box 9, folder 28: "Brochures/Factsheets/ Publications: Publication: *Lesbian Health Activism: The First Wave,* 2001," Records of the Mautner Project, Schlesinger. This document, reproduced in *Lesbian Health Activism,* was originally from *Our Bodies, Ourselves.* Mary O'Donnell, "Lesbian Health Care: Issues and Literature," in *Lesbian Health Activism: The First Wave; Feminist Writings from the Early Lesbian Health Movement,* December 1973, Feminist Health Press, box 9, folder 28: "Brochures/Factsheets/ Publications: Publication: *Lesbian Health Activism: The First Wave,* 2001," Records of the Mautner Project, Schlesinger.

Notes to Chapter 3

Epigraph: Frankfort, *Vaginal Politics,* xiii–xiv.

1 See Keane, "Second-Wave Feminism in the American South," where she argues that feminist clinics did not view this as co-optation. Rather, they saw reforming mainstream institutions as central to their mission.
2 Price, "The Self Help Clinic."
3 Silliman et al., *Undivided Rights*; Nelson, *Women of Color and the Reproductive Rights Movement*; Nelson, *More Than Medicine.*
4 Feminist Women's Health Center, "Update on Harvey Karman," April 20, 1974, box 15, folder 2: "[Feminist Women's Health Center, Los Angeles]: Karman, Harvey, 1974–1976, n.d.," WCHCR, Schlesinger.
5 Fran Moira, "Infighting? Or Righteous Law-Breaking," *off our backs,* July 31, 1975, 24.
6 Dorothy Townsend, "Vigilantes Claim It Was Illegal: Militant Feminists Raid L.A. Abortion Unit," *Los Angeles Times,* September, 4, 1974, box 15, folder 2: "[Feminist Women's Health Center, Los Angeles]: Karman, Harvey, 1974–1976, n.d.," WCHCR, Schlesinger.
7 "Hearing for a Preliminary Injunction: Women's Community Service Center vs. Feminist Women's Health Center," September 30, 1974, box 15, folder 2: "[Feminist Women's Health Center, Los Angeles]: Karman, Harvey, 1974–1976, n.d.," WCHCR, Schlesinger.
8 Emphasis in original. Barbara Orrok to Burt Pines, April 30, 1975, box 15, folder 2: "[Feminist Women's Health Center, Los Angeles]: Karman, Harvey, 1974–1976, n.d.," WCHCR, Schlesinger.
9 Quoted in Moira, "Infighting?," 24.
10 Margaret Sanger founded the American Birth Control League, which later became Planned Parenthood. This U.S. organization is now part of a larger one, the International Planned Parenthood Federation.
11 "History and Successes," Planned Parenthood, accessed March 22, 2012, http:// www.plannedparenthood.org/about-us/who-we-are/history-and-successes.htm.
12 Banzhaf interview, 2015.
13 Jill Benderly, "Does Corporate Giant Fill Health Care Needs Like Feminist Clinics?," *Women and Health,* January/February 1990, box 52, folder: "Planned Parenthood of Greater Iowa, The Source, 1990 and 1994," EGCR, IWA.

14 Banzhaf interview, 2015.

15 Banzhaf interview, 2015.

16 Feminist Women's Health Center, "Controversies in Birth Control," July 19, 1978, box 6, folder: "Women's Health in Women's Hands (2 of 9)," FWHCR, SBC.

17 Farber and Law did not report whether the guard threw them out on the orders of APPP or not. Feminist Women's Health Center, "Remember Margaret!," April 17, 1975, carton 3, folder 145: "Feminist Women's Health Center (Los Angeles)," BSP, Schlesinger. Self-help activists were not alone in lodging complaints against Planned Parenthood, and these complaints did not end in the 1970s. Members of the women's health movement and the reproductive rights movement, whose efforts focused more on lobbying for legislation, had been making demands of mainstream medical institutions for years. For example, in 1981 the Reproductive Rights National Network called Planned Parenthood "the best example of an international population control organization that successfully maintains a benevolent, 'woman-helping' image in the U.S." Reproductive Rights National Network, "Rough Road Ahead," *off our backs*, August/Semptember 1981, 10, 17.

18 The list of demands did not specify which contraceptives they were concerned about.

19 Feminist Women's Health Center, "Remember Margaret!"

20 Ironically, "siege" was a term pro-choice activists usually reserved for anti-abortion activism.

21 "Woman Controlled Clinic Meeting," April 3, 1989, box 24, folder 3: "Reproductive Rights, 1981–84, n.d.," NWHNR, SSC.

22 Benderly, "Does Corporate Giant Fill Health Care Needs Like Feminist Clinics?"

23 "Woman Controlled Clinic Meeting."

24 Dana M. Gallagher to Norma Swenson, May 7, 1989, box 24, folder 3: "Reproductive Rights, 1981–84, n.d.," NWHNR, SSC.

25 Women's Community Health Center, "Self-Help as an Organizing Tool."

26 See Hans A. Baer, *Biomedicine and Alternative Healing Systems in America: Issues of Class, Race, Ethnicity, and Gender* (Madison: University of Wisconsin Press, 2001).

27 Jessica Lipnack, "A Special Report: The Women's Health Movement," *New Age*, box 1, folder 9: "Articles, 1979–99," NWHNR, SSC.

28 Eubank, "The Speculum and the Cul-de-Sac," 132.

29 Martha Shelley, "What Is FEN?," 1976, box 1, folder: "FEN (Feminist Economic Network), 1976," DFWHCR, WPRL.

30 Kathy McManus, "Practicing at Medicine," *New West*, April 1981, box 47, folder 9: "Collaborations. Feminist Women's Health Center, Los Angeles, California [transcript of meeting following August 25, 1976, meeting of Abortion League; newsletters, clippings, etc., 1981]," BWHBC, Schlesinger.

31 "Full-Time Staff" to "Monday Night Meeting," box 13, folder: "General Minutes, January 1973–September 1974," EGCR, IWA.

32 "Meeting with Dick," March 4, 1976, box 13, folder: "Doctors' Committee, 1975–1978, 1980," EGCR, IWA.

33 The archival records from this particular clinic require users to keep staff members' names anonymous, so Susan Miller and Peter North are pseudonyms.

34 Deb, "C/SC for Meeting with Dick," April 15, 1976, box 13, folder: "Doctors' Committee, 1975–1978, 1980," EGCR, IWA.

35 Adele to Ab Committee, box 13, folder: "Doctors' Committee, 1975–1978, 1980," EGCR, IWA.

36 "Doctor's Committee," June 17, 1977, box 13, folder: "Doctors' Committee, 1975–1978, 1980," EGCR, IWA.

37 Keane, "Second-Wave Feminism in the American South"; Banzhaf interview, 2015; Hornstein interview 2015; Tallahassee Feminist Women's Health Center, "Anti-trust Suit Settlement!!!," *The Examiner*, April 1980, 1–4, box 47, folder 10: "Collaborations, Feminist Women's Health Center, Tallahassee, Florida, 1975–1980," BWHBCR, Schlesinger.

38 Keane, "Second-Wave Feminism in the American South," 212–213.

39 Lolly Hirsch and Jeanne Hirsch, "Update of the Tallahassee Feminist Women's Health Center Trial," *Monthly Extract* 5:3 (1976): 4.

40 *Feminist Women's Health Center, Inc., a Florida Non-profit Corporation, v. Mahmood Mohammad, M.D. et al.*, Justia U.S. Law, accessed March 22, 2012, http://law.justia.com/cases/federal/appellate-courts/F2/586/530/291524/.

41 Feminist Women's Health Center, press release, October 1, 1975, carton 3, folder 145: "Feminist Women's Health Center (Los Angeles, Tallahassee), 1971–1978," BSP, Schlesinger.

42 Brian Richardson, "Medical Clinic Suit Dismissed," *Tallahassee Democrat*, December 21, 1976, 21, box 18, folder 6: "WATCH, 1976–1978," WCHCR, Schlesinger.

43 Hirsch and Hirsch, "Update of the Tallahassee Feminist Women's Health Center Trial."

44 Richardson, "Medical Clinic Suit Dismissed."

45 Tallahassee Feminist Women's Health Center, "Anti-trust Suit Settlement!!!"

46 *Goldfarb v. Virginia State Bar*, 94 F.T.C. at 1005–06.

47 Women Acting Together to Combat Harassment, "WATCH Information," box 4, folder 4: "Grants: Already Written, 1974–1980, n.d.," WCHCR, Schlesinger.

48 Keane, "Second-Wave Feminism in the American South," 212–213.

49 "Who Controls Birthing: WATCH Battle," *Feminist Women's Health Center Review*, December 1979, box 15, folder 6: "Feminist Women's Health Center, Santa Ana, Calif., 1974–1979," WCHCR, Schlesinger.

50 Women Acting Together to Combat Harassment, "WATCH Information."

51 Jacqueline H. Wolf, *Deliver Me from Pain: Anesthesia and Birth in America* (Baltimore: Johns Hopkins University Press, 2011), 185–186.

52 "Factsheet: Four Women Arrested in Florida, Childbirth Practices Challenged," 1977, box 2, folder 57: MOTHER (Mothers of the wHole Earth Revolt)," DFWHCR, WPRL.

53 Women Acting Together to Combat Harassment, "WATCH Information."

54 Becky Chalker suggested that only these four were arrested because they were the only ones that hospital personnel recognized in order to report them. Rebecca Chalker, interview by Hannah Dudley-Shotwell, March 19, 2015.

55 Quoted in Keane, "Second-Wave Feminism in the American South," 220. The local TV station manager confiscated the film, but it is unclear why. In response, the WATCH members asked, "What information does [the hospital] fear? If hospital administrators had nothing to fear, this film would have been aired without any problem." See Women Acting Together to Combat Harassment, "WATCH Information."

56 "Health Activists 'Inspect' Maternity Ward, Go to Jail," *Ob/Gyn News*, October 17, 1977, 2, box 18, folder 6: "WATCH, 1976–1978," WCHCR, Schlesinger.

57 WATCH to Friends of WATCH, June 1, 1977, box 18, folder 6: "WATCH, 1976–1978," WCHCR, Schlesinger.

58 WATCH, "Feminists Railroaded in Tallahassee Trespass Case," box 18, folder 6: "WATCH, 1976–1978," WCHCR, Schlesinger.

59 Wendy Kline, "'Please Include This in Your Book': Readers Respond to *Our Bodies, Ourselves*," *Bulletin of the History of Medicine* 79:1 (2005): 81–110; W. Kline, *Bodies of Knowledge*. Kline gives an excellent full chapter account of the PTP. I recount much the same story here briefly in order to put it in the context of other self-help activism.

60 Susan Bell, "Political Gynecology: Gynecological Imperialism and the Politics of Self-Help," *Science for the People*, September-October 1979, 8–14, box 25, folder 10: "Self-Help OB/GYN, 1979–94, n.d.," Native American Women's Health Education Resource Center Records (hereafter NAWHERCR), SSC. As Kline notes, medical students of the 1970s were not immune to the influence of healthcare reform. Particularly as the proportion of women in these programs increased, many medical students "engaged in political protests, demanded that their schools respond to the local community's health needs, and promoted educational reform." W. Kline, *Bodies of Knowledge*, 45.

61 Pelvic Teaching Group, "Position Paper," June 1976, box 12, folder 7: "Pelvic Teaching Program: Correspondence with Medical Schools," WCHCR, Schlesinger.

62 Bell, "Political Gynecology," NAWHERCR, SSC.

63 Bell; W. Kline, *Bodies of Knowledge*.

64 Pelvic Teaching Group, "Position Paper."

65 Bell, "Political Gynecology," NAWHERCR, SSC.

66 Bell, "Political Gynecology." The PTP was not alone in their frustrations; some self-help activists feared "being used as cheap labor" by the medical system. Some had noticed a trend of local doctors scheduling a checkup with women and then sending them to feminist clinics for diaphragm fittings, for example. The fitting and the explanation of how to use the diaphragm took about an hour and a half, which was much longer than most doctors were willing to work with a patient. Self-help activists feared that both the doctors and the clients saw them as just "nice nurses" cooperating with the medical system. This trend of being used by the medical system prompted many self-help groups to rethink their strategies. Even though the PTP ended, trainings like it did not disappear altogether. Since the 1970s, programs like the PTP have spread to at least half of all U.S. medical schools. Some hospitals now employ pelvic teaching models to train nurses for positions as sexual assault forensics examiners (SAFEs), who do compassionate evidence collection exams for rape survivors. See "At Your Cervix: A Documentary," accessed December 29, 2015, http://atyourcervixmovie.com/gtas.shtml. In many places, the program has also expanded to include men who, for example, model for urology exams. However, most models are not self-help activists; doctors often train them. The programs certainly are not as self-help-based as PTP members wanted in the 1970s, but they do offer a glimpse into the lasting impact of self-help activists' success at impacting mainstream medicine in both the United States and Europe. Erin St. John Kelly, "Teaching Doctors Sensitivity on the Most Sensitive of Exams," *New York Times*, June 2, 1998, http://www.nytimes

.com/1998/06/02/science/teaching-doctors-sensitivity-on-the-most-sensitive-of
-exams.html?pagewanted=all. International studies have shown that students who
learn from pelvic teaching models are more knowledgeable and more comfortable
with the exams. Kjell Wanggren et al., "Teaching Medical Students Gynaecological Examination Using Professional Patients: Evaluation of Students' Skills and
Feelings," *Medical Teacher* 27:2 (2005): 130–135; Women's Community Health
Center, "A Report from Women's Community Health Center," 13.

67 Pelvic Teaching Group, "Position Paper." Emphasis in original.

Notes to Chapter 4

Epigraph: Fran Moira, "reading right to keep fit," *off our backs* 11:8, (August |
September, 1981): 22.

1 Rosalyn Baxandall and Linda Gordon, introduction to *Dear Sisters: Dispatches
from the Women's Liberation Movement* (New York: Basic Books, 2000), 20. Anne
Valk, "Living a Feminist Lifestyle: The Intersection of Theory and Action in a
Lesbian Feminist Collective," in Hewitt, *No Permanent Waves: Recasting
Histories of U.S. Feminism*, ed. Nancy Hewitt (New Brunswick, NJ: Rutgers
University Press, 2010).

2 Most cervical cap providers ordered caps from Europe, because they were not
manufactured in the United States.

3 "The Cervical Cap," box 32, folder: "Cervical Cap Studies," FWHCR, SBC.

4 Emma Goldman Clinic, "The Cervical Cap Handbook for Fitters and Users," 1981,
box 30, folder: "Cervical Cap Handbook, 1981, 1988 and undated," EGCR, IWA.

5 He noted that the lemon juice worked as a spermicide as well. Mary-Sherman
Willis, "Cervical Caps: Old and Yet Too New," *Science News*, December 22 and
29, 1979, box 27, folder 2, "Subject Files: Cervical Cap, 1979–1992," BWHBC,
Additional Records, Schlesinger; Emma Goldman Clinic, "The Cervical Cap
Handbook for Fitters and Users." Over the next several decades, women and their
physicians also began using the cap as an aid to conception. In 1950, Dr. M. J.
Whitelaw published an article in *Fertility and Sterility* describing how he used
"a plastic cervical cap filled with the husband's semen applied to the cervix for
24 hours" in order to help a couple become pregnant. Other physicians followed
suit. W. J. Whitelaw, "Use of the Cervical Cap to Increase Fertility in Case of
Oligospermia," *Fertility and Sterility* 1:1 (1950): 33–39.

6 Gina Kolata, "The Sad Legacy of the Dalkon Shield," *New York Times*, December 6, 1987, http://www.nytimes.com/1987/12/06/magazine/the-sad-legacy-of-the
-dalkon-shield.html; Clare L. Roepke and Eric A. Schaff, "Long Tail Strings:
Impact of the Dalkon Shield 40 Years Later," *Open Journal of Obstetrics and
Gynecology* 4 (2014): 996–1005.

7 In 1978, prescriptions for diaphragms increased nearly 140 percent. Rebecca
Chalker, *Complete Cervical Cap Guide* (New York: Harper and Row, 1987).

8 Rebecca Chalker, email correspondence with Hannah Dudley-Shotwell,
August 13, 2015.

9 Several members of the women's health movement became interested in the cap as
a method of contraception in the mid-1970s. Health activist and author Barbara
Seaman encountered the cervical cap in Europe in the mid-1970s and included a
chapter on its use in her 1977 book, *Women and the Crisis in Sex Hormones* (New

York: Bantam Books, 1977). Around the same time, Irene Snair, a nurse practitioner at the Student Health Service at New England College, read about the cap in a textbook and wrote to Lamberts, the company that sold them in Europe, for more information. She ordered several and began fitting them at the Student Health Service. Snair fit nursing student Sarah Berndt with a cap, and Berndt introduced it to the women she worked with part-time at the New Hampshire Feminist Health Center. In 1978, *Our Bodies, Ourselves* published an article on the cap and distributed it widely among women's health activists around the United States. As a result of the Dalkon Shield crisis in 1976, Congress amended the Federal Food, Drug, and Cosmetics Act to include regulations on medical devices. It developed three classes of devices: Class I were devices with the lowest risk, and Class III devices held the highest risk. The FDA classified caps used for the purposes of artificial insemination as Class II and caps used for the purposes of contraception as Class III, ruling that, if used in this manner, the cap posed "significant risk" to users. Many cap providers learned of the new classification in 1980, when the FDA ordered all cap shipments into the United States to be seized at entry ports. Cervical cap proponents argued that choosing a form of contraception was always a form of risk-taking, and that as long as a woman understood the risk, she should be free to choose any method available. They also argued that this method was significantly less risky than many of the other methods available to women, including the Pill and the IUD. Chalker, *The Complete Cervical Cap Guide.*

10 Dana Gallagher and Gary Richwald, "Feminism and Regulation Collide: The Food and Drug Administration's Approval of the Cervical Cap," *Women and Health* 15 (2009): 87–97.

11 The groups included Yakima Feminist Women's Health Center in Yakima, Washington; Everywoman's Clinic in San Francisco, California; Portland Women's Health Center in Portland, Oregon; and five Federation of Feminist Women's Health Center Clinics: Atlanta Feminist Women's Health Center in Atlanta, Georgia; Los Angeles Feminist Women's Health Center in Los Angeles, California; Orange County Feminist Women's Health Center in Santa Ana, California; Chico Feminist Women's Health Center in Chico, California; and Womancare in San Diego, California. See "The Cervical Cap," FWHCR, SBC.

12 Loie Sauer, "Cervical Cap, a Contraceptive, Emerges as an 'Attractive' Option," *New York Times,* August 26, 1980, box 27, folder 2: "Cervical Cap, 1979–1992," BWHBC, Additional Records, Schlesinger.

13 "The Cervical Cap," FWHCR, SBC

14 "Cervical Cap Parties," *Newsletter of the Feminist Women's Health Center,* September 1981, box 47, folder 9: "Collaborations. Feminist Women's Health Center, Los Angeles, California [transcript of meeting following August 25, 1976, meeting of Abortion League; newsletters, clippings, etc., 1981]," BWHBC, Schlesinger.

15 Banzhaf interview, 2015.

16 Bread and Roses Women's Health Center, Inc., box 32, folder: "Fitting, Models and Problems," EGCR, IWA.

17 "The Cervical Cap," FWHCR, SBC.

18 Lorraine Rothman, "The Cervical Cap and the FDA: Safety and Efficacy for Whom?," box 55, folder 15,Toni Carabillo and Judith Meuli Papers (hereafter Carabillo and Meuli Papers), Schlesinger; "Cervical Cap," Planned Parenthood, http://www.plannedparenthood.org/learn/birth-control/cervical-cap.

19 "Model Preparation Meeting," box 32, folder: "Fitting, Models, and Problems," EGCR, IWA.

20 Chalker interview, 2015.

21 In the late 1980s, the FDA withdrew approval of most forms of the cap, citing the possibility of vaginal lacerations and irritation. Since that time, new cervical cap brands have hit the market and are offered on a limited basis in the United States today. "Cervical Cap," Planned Parenthood.

22 These practices go by a variety of names, including OM, Billings Method, natural family planning, natural birth control, the cervical mucus method, and fertility consciousness.

23 "Northeast Alliance—Founding Weekend, October 27–29, 1978, Peterborough, New Hampshire," box 13, folder 9: "Rising Sun Feminist Health Alliance Mailings and Notes, 1978–1979," BWHBC, Additional Records, Schlesinger; Jessica Lipnack and Jeffrey Stamps, *Networking, the First Report and Directory* (Garden City, NY: Doubleday, 1982), 21.

24 Susan Bell et al., "Reclaiming Reproductive Control: A Feminist Approach to Fertility Consciousness," *Science for the People*, January/February 1980, 6–35, box 214, folder 9: "Natural Birth Control, 1979–85, n.d.," NWHNR, SSC.

25 Rising Sun Feminist Health Alliance, meeting minutes, January 27–29, 1979, box 13, folder 9: "Rising Sun Feminist Health Alliance Mailings and Notes," BWHBC, Additional Records, Schlesinger.

26 Bell et al., "Reclaiming Reproductive Control."

27 Susan Bell, "Feminist Self-Help: The Case of Fertility Consciousness / Women Controlled Natural Birth Control Groups," box 47, folder: "Natural Methods of Family Planning, 1982–93," Loretta J. Ross Papers, SSC.

28 Helen Holmes, Betty Hoskins, and Michael Gross, *Birth Control and Controlling Birth: Women-Centered Perspectives* (Clifton, NJ: Humana Press, 1980), 78.

29 Suzann Gage, "Sexuality: Donor Insemination," *Lesbian News*, August 1985, in *Lesbian Health Activism: The First Wave; Feminist Writings from the Early Lesbian Health Movement*, December 1973, Feminist Health Press, box 9, folder 28: "Brochures/Factsheets/Publications: Publication: *Lesbian Health Activism: The First Wave*, 2001," Records of the Mautner Project, Schlesinger.

30 "Fertility Consciousness and Woman-Controlled Natural Birth Control," box 12, folder 5: "Ovulation Method / Women Controlled Birth Control Self-Help Group, 1978–1979, n.d.," WCHCR, Schlesinger.

31 WCHC files did not yield any evidence that the group responded to Billings. John Billings to "The President, Fertility Consciousness Programme, Women's Community Health Centre," October 11, 1979, box 30, folder: "Subject Files: Natural Birth Control, 1975–1997," BWHBC, Additional Records, Schlesinger.

32 Holmes, Hoskins, and Gross, *Birth Control and Controlling Birth*, 77.

33 Holmes, Hoskins, and Gross, 71.

34 Holmes, Hoskins, and Gross, 77–78.

35 Hornstein interview, 2018.

36 Francie Hornstein, "Children by Donor Insemination: A New Choice for Lesbians," in *Test Tube Women: What Future for Motherhood?*, ed. Rita Arditti, Renate Duelli Klein, and Shelley Minden (Boston: Pandora Press, 1984), 374; Gage, "Sexuality."

37 Laura Mamo, *Queering Reproduction: Achieving Pregnancy in the Age of Technoscience* (Durham, NC: Duke University Press, 2007).

38 Yael Peskin, interview by Hannah Dudley-Shotwell and Gill Frank, June 25, 2018.

39 For an account of self-help donor insemination in the UK, see Renate Duelli Klein, "Doing It Ourselves: Self Insemination," in *Test Tube Women: What Future for Motherhood?*, ed. Rita Arditti, Renate Duelli Klein, and Shelley Minden (Boston: Pandora Press, 1984), 382–390.

40 R. H. Foote, "The History of Artificial Insemination: Selected Notes and Notables," *American Society of Animal Science*, 2002, accessed December 29, 2015, https://www.asas.org/docs/publications/footehist.pdf?sfvrsn=0.

41 Peskin interview, 2018.

42 Hornstein interview, 2018.

43 Hornstein interview, 2018.

44 Hornstein interview, 2015. Four years later, Peskin also got pregnant the same way with the same donor.

45 Hornstein, "Children by Donor Insemination," 374.

46 R. Klein, "Doing It Ourselves," 382–384; Gage, "Sexuality."

47 Hornstein interview, 2018.

48 Gage, "Sexuality." Because sperm banks would only sell to certain women (read: married and heterosexual), several woman-controlled clinics began purchasing sperm themselves and selling it to their clients. Hornstein, "Children by Donor Insemination," 376–377; Chalker interview, 2015. Some of these clinics that remained open (the Atlanta FWHC, for example) still offer donor insemination services today. Rising Sun members also considered setting up their own informal network of sperm donors, but the plan did not come to fruition. Rising Sun Feminist Health Alliance, meeting minutes, January 27–29, 1979. In subsequent decades, sperm banks have altered their policies and do not discriminate based on sexuality or marital status. However, almost all are unwilling to sell sperm to women without the signature of a licensed physician. Only New York and Georgia have state laws that require physician consent for a woman to purchase sperm. Many sperm banks have implemented these policies on their own. The one exception I have found in the United States is Northwest Cryobank in Washington State.

49 Peskin interview, 2018.

50 Amy Agigian, *Baby Steps: How Lesbian Alternative Insemination Is Changing the World* (Middletown, CT: Wesleyan University Press, 2004), 5.

51 Karren Kowalski, ed., *Nursing Dimensions* 3(1): 73–77, carton 1, folder: "Women's Newsletter and Periodical Collection."

52 Rosetta Reitz, *Menopause: A Positive Approach* (New York: Penguin Books, 1977), 96–97.

53 Reitz.

54 In the 1980s, groups such as the Older Women's League (OWL) worked to address the economic impact of aging and the limitations of older women's access to medical care. See Patricia Huckle, *Tish Sommers, Activist, and the Founding of the Older Women's League* (Knoxville: University of Tennessee Press, 1991); Judith Houck, *Hot and Bothered: Women, Medicine, and Menopause in Modern America* (Cambridge: Harvard University Press, 2008).

55 The San Francisco Women's Health Collective, the Berkeley Women's Health Collective, and the Cambridge Women's Community Health Center all had active groups.

56 Kathleen MacPherson, "Hot Flash!! Women Reclaim Menopause," *Sojourner*,

February 1981, 11, box 21, folder 17: "Midlife and Older Women, 1982–84," NWHNR, SSC.

57 Quoted in MacPherson, 11.

58 Louise Corbett, "Getting Our Bodies Back: Menopausal Self-Help Groups," box 21, folder 17: "Midlife and Older Women, 1982–84," NWHNR, SSC.

59 MacPherson, "Feminist Praxis in the Making," 225–229. MacPherson was deeply aware that her role as both researcher and Menopause Collective member also added another layer to the already fraught group dynamic; she deals carefully with this issue in the first chapter of her dissertation.

60 The group mailed over nine hundred packets of information on menopause and self-help to "most states in the union." They decided that they should send only materials written by group members or by other women with a "feminist perspective." They eliminated all articles written by a male doctor from their packet. MacPherson, "Feminist Praxis in the Making," 300–303.

61 MacPherson, 232–277.

62 MacPherson, 348–363; Davi Birnbaum, "Mid-life Women," *Network News*, January/February 1983, box 1, folder 2: "Annual Reports, 1977–2006," NWHNR, SSC; National Women's Health Network, "Network Committees," box 21, folder 17: "Midlife and Older Women, 1982–1984," NWHNR, SSC; Wanda Wooten, "Midlife and Older Women's Health Project Proposal Draft (2nd)," January 11, 1983, box 45, folder 6: "Midlife and Older Women's Project," NWHNR, SSC; National Women's Health Network, "Empowering Mid-life and Older Women to Enhance Their Later Years," box 21, folder 17: "Midlife and Older Women, 1982–84," NWHNR, SSC.

63 MacPherson, "Feminist Praxis in the Making," 408–409.

64 MacPherson, 59–62.

65 MacPherson, 46.

66 MacPherson.

67 MacPherson, 363.

68 MacPherson.

69 MacPherson, 387.

70 MacPherson, 278–298.

71 Fran Moira, "Health Reviews: Reading Right to Keep Fit," *off our backs* 11:8 (1981): 22.

Notes to Chapter 5

1 James P. Rife and Alan J. Dellapenna, *Caring and Curing: A History of the Indian Health Service* (Terra Alta, WV: PHS Commissioner Officers Foundation for the Advancement of Public Health, 2009); Gurr, *Reproductive Justice: The Politics of Health Care for Native American Women* (New Brunswick, NJ: Rutgers University Press, 2015); A. Smith, *Conquest: Sexual Violence and American Indian Genocide* (Cambridge, MA: South End Press, 2005).

2 Nelson, *More Than Medicine: Sexual Violence and American Indian Genocide* (Cambridge, MA: South End Press, 2005), 163.

3 In seeking a way to differentiate self-help as practiced by groups such as the NBWHP from gynecological self-help, I asked prominent NBWHP leaders Loretta Ross and Byllye Avery what term they would apply to this particular brand of self-help. Each offered "psychological" as the best epithet, even though

this group and related ones typically just used "self-help" on its own to describe their activities. For the sake of clarity, I use "psychological self-help" whenever I need to distinguish their activities from "gynecological self-help." Many other groups of women also developed their own unique uses for self-help. For example, the National Latina Health Organization adapted the NBWHP's psychological self-help model to suit their own needs, tackling issues such as teenage self-esteem and local violence. Other multiracial groups, including the SisterSong Women of Color Reproductive Justice Collective, SisterLove, and Be Present Inc., developed self-help processes as a way for women to dialogue in coalitions. These groups mostly developed in the late 1980s and 1990s, and all of them continued their self-help activities into the twenty-first century.

4   Health activist and scholar Loretta Ross argued that "women of color" was useful as a term of solidarity and because it was a term that women of color created, rather than a term imposed upon them. I use the term when a group used it to refer to themselves. (The NBWHP, SisterSong, SisterLove, and Be Present, Inc. use the term frequently in their literature.) See "Origin of the Phrase 'Women of Color,'" YouTube video, 2:59, posted by Western States Center, February 15, 2011, https://www.youtube.com/watch?v=82vl34mi4Iw.

5   Scholars and activists who examine women of color's and indigenous women's self-help-based organizations include Silliman et al., *Undivided Rights: Women of Color Organize for Reproductive Justice* (Cambridge, MA: South End Press, 2004); Nelson, *More Than Medicine*; Jennifer Nelson, "'All This That Has Happened to Me Shouldn't Happen to Nobody Else': Loretta Ross and the Women of Color Reproductive Freedom Movement of the 1980s," *Journal of Women's History* 22:3 (2010): 136–160; Charon Asetoyer, Katharine Cronk, and Samanthi Hewakapuge, *Indigenous Women's Health Book, within the Sacred Circle: Reproductive Rights, Environmental Health, Traditional Herbs and Remedies* (Lake Andes, SD: Pine Hill Press, 2003); Evan Hart, "Building a More Inclusive Women's Health Movement: Byllye Avery and the Development of the National Black Women's Health Project, 1981–1990" (PhD diss., University of Cincinnati, 2012); Morgen, *Into Our Own Hands: The Women's Health Movement in the United States, 1969–1990* (New Brunswick, NJ: Rutgers University Press, 2002).

6   Nelson, *Women of Color and the Reproductive Rights Movement*; Silliman et al., *Undivided Rights*; D. Roberts, *Killing the Black Body: Race, Reproduction, and the Meaning of Liberty* (New York: Pantheon Books, 1997); L. Ross et al., *Radical Reproductive Justice: An Introduction* (Oakland: University of California Press, 2017).

7   SisterSong Women of Color Reproductive Justice Collective, "What Is RJ?," accessed March 31, 2015, http://sistersong.net/index.php?option=com _content&view=article&id=141&Itemid=8; L. Ross et al., *Radical Reproductive Justice*.

8   "Power: Rx for Good Health," *Ms. Magazine*, May 1986, 56–62, box 104, folder 2: "Women's Health: The Press and Public Policy, 2005," NWHNR, SSC.

9   Avery interview, 2005, 15.

10   Avery interview, 2005, 16–19.

11   Birth and Wellness Center of Gainesville, accessed December 1, 2015, http://birthwellnessofgainesville.com/home/.

12   Silliman et al., *Undivided Rights*, 66; Avery interview, 2005, 24.

13   The original name of the organization was the National Women's Health Lobby. Silliman et al., *Undivided Rights*, 34.

14 "Power: Rx for Good Health."

15 On the "conspiracy of silence," see Patricia Hill Collins, *Black Feminist Thought: Knowledge, Consciousness, and the Politics of Empowerment* (Boston: Unwin Hyman, 1990). The BWHP would later become the National Black Women's Health Project (NBWHP).

16 Linda Villarosa, *Body and Soul: The Black Women's Guide to Physical Health and Emotional Well-Being* (New York: Harper Perennial, 1994), xv; "Power: Rx for Good Health."

17 Avery interview, 2005, 25–26.

18 As part of her graduate program, Allen learned about a variety of therapeutic approaches to deal with negative emotions, but she felt that none of them would fully enable her to develop a positive "sense of self." One such therapeutic program that Allen encountered was Re-evaluation Counseling (RC). In RC support groups, one person at a time was the center of attention. The group allowed this person space to "discharge" emotion. While Allen liked the idea of this process because it was useful for thinking through one's feelings, she also thought it was not results-oriented, and there was no emphasis on what to do about negative feelings or how to turn them into actions. She thought that participants got stuck in the "navel gazing" and did not move forward to turn their pain and healing into political activism. Allen felt that programs like RC should have a political component. Further, very few African Americans participated in RC, and this model did not focus on racial issues. Lillie Allen, interview by Loretta Ross, 2003. Several historians credit Allen's training in Re-evaluation Counseling as the stimulus for creating the self-help model practiced by the NBWHP. In a personal conversation, she stated that she was influenced by a variety of therapeutic models. Silliman et al., *Undivided Rights*, 69; Loretta Ross, Voices of Feminism Oral History Project, interview by Joyce Follet, 2004–2005, 204–205.

19 Ross interview, 2004–2005, 203–205.

20 Hart, "Building a More Inclusive Women's Health Movement," 61.

21 Loretta Ross, interview by Hannah Dudley-Shotwell, August 18, 2015; Hart, "Building a More Inclusive Women's Health Movement."

22 Julie Rioux, "Black Women's Health: Empowerment through Wellness," *Gay Community News*, February 25–March 3, 1990, box 26, folder 1: "Women of Color and Health, 1990–98, n.d.," NAWHERCR, SSC.

23 Ross interview, 2004–2005; "Black and Female: What Is the Reality?," February 15, 1988, 46, box 104, folder 1: "Allies Training, 1988," NWHNR, SSC.

24 "PR Plan for the Black Women's Health Project," box 104, folder 6: "Black Women's Health Conference, 1983, Funding and Budgets, 1983," NWHNR, SSC.

25 Avery interview, 2005, 32–33.

26 Byllye Avery, funding application to the Funding Exchange; "Black Women's Health Project/Conference," September 15, 1982, box 104, folder 7: "Black Women's Health Conference, 1983, Schedules, Programs, and Printed Material, 1982–83," NWHNR, SSC.

27 Hart, "Building a More Inclusive Women's Health Movement," 65.

28 Avery, funding application to the Funding Exchange.

29 Belita Cowan and Byllye Avery, "Black Women's Self-Help Study Groups in Georgia, North Carolina, and South Carolina," National Black Women's Health Project / National Women's Health Network, funding application to the Fund for Southern Communities, box 104, folder 13: "Grant Proposals and Related Correspondence, 1981–83, n.d.," NWHNR, SSC.

30 Quoted in Betty Norwood Chaney, "Black Women's Health Conference," *Southern Changes* 5 (1983): 18–20, http://southernchanges.digitalscholarship .emory.edu/sco5-5_1204/sco5-5_008/.

31 Hart, "Building a More Inclusive Women's Health Movement," 60.

32 Avery interview, 2005, 26–29.

33 "Power: Rx for Good Health."

34 Chaney, "Black Women's Health Conference."

35 Ross interview, 2004–2005, 203.

36 Felicia Ward, "I Met Lillie . . . and Discovered Myself, or How Self-Help Programmes Are Born," August 1987, box 17, folder 3: "Annual Meetings, 1988–89," Ross Papers, SSC.

37 National Black Women's Health Project, "Open Your Life," box 17, folder 10: "Promotional Material," Ross Papers, SSC.

38 Maureen Downey, "A Healthy Concern for Black Women: Crisis of 'Being Sick and Tired' Gave Birth to Feminist's Projects," *Atlanta Journal-Constitution*, May 7, 1987.

39 Ward, "I Met Lillie."

40 Ross interview, 2004–2005, 206.

41 Ross interview, 2015.

42 L. Ross et al., *Radical Reproductive Justice*.

43 "Black and Female: What Is the Reality?"

44 Avery interview, 2005, 30; Peter Scott, "Community: The Atlanta Project Clusters—Center's Potpourri of Services Cater to Black Women's Health," *Atlanta Journal -Constitution*, June 30, 1994, N10; National Black Women's Health Project, "Targeted Program Development: Public Housing, Context for Change the Center for Black Women's Wellness," box 19, folder 2: "Empowerment through Wellness, 1989," Ross Papers, SSC. Byllye Avery, "A Proposal for General Support of the Black Women's Health Project, National Women's Health Network," December 1983, 8–9, box 104, folder 13: "Grant Proposals and Related Correspondence, 1981–83, n.d.," NWHNR, SSC.

45 Avery, "A Proposal for General Support of the Black Women's Health Project."

46 Some scholars use the term "mutual aid" to refer to self-help groups more broadly. In particular, this term often denotes eighteenth- and nineteenth-century Friendly Societies and craft guilds and so forth, but can also refer to twentieth-century iterations of voluntary reciprocal exchange groups like the self-help groups of the women's health movement. See David T. Beito, *From Mutual Aid to the Welfare State: Fraternal Societies and Social Services, 1890—1967* (Chapel Hill: University of North Carolina Press, 2000), 1–2.

47 National Black Women's Health Project, "Self-Help Program Process," box 19, folder 2: "Empowerment through Wellness, 1989," Ross Papers, SSC.

48 Rosenbaum, "Whose Bodies? Whose Selves?," 122.

49 Avery interview, 2005, 30–31.

50 Downey, "A Healthy Concern for Black Women"; Andrea Rivera-Cano, foreword to *Contact: A Bimonthly Publication of the Christian Medical Commission World Council of Churches* 98 (August 1987), box 17, folder 3: "Annual Meetings, 1988–89," Ross Papers, SSC.

51 "NBWHP Guide to Self-Help Group Development," *National Black Women's Health Project Self-Help Developers' Manual*, 10–11(1990), box #09S-83 (unprocessed), Black Women's Health Imperiative Records (hereafter BWHIR), SSC; "A

Good Self-Help Group Is a Mutual Self-Help Process" box 17, folder 10: "NBWHP, Organizational Materials, Promotional Material, 1985–1987, n.d.," Ross Papers, SSC.

52 These women included Loretta Ross, Mary Lisbon, Faye Williams, Ajowa Ifateyo, and Linda Leaks. Ross often distinguished between gynecological self-help and Allen's form of self-help by calling the former "drop your pants" self-help. Ross interview, 2004–2005, 206; Ross interview, 2015. In 1993, the NBWHP created a video titled *It's OK to Peek* giving women instructions on how to do cervical self-exam.

53 This award is given annually to about twenty to thirty Americans who the MacArthur Foundation believes are doing exceptional work in their field. MacArthur Foundation, accessed January 15, 2016, https://www.macfound.org/.

54 Ross interview, 2004–2005, 206.

55 Ross interview, 2004–2005, 208.

56 "Self-Help Program Description," box 17, folder 3: "Annual Meetings, 1988–89," Ross Papers, SSC.

57 "Self-Help Program Description."

58 Ross interview, 2015.

59 "Power: Rx for Good Health."

60 Chaney, "Black Women's Health Conference."

61 Scott, "Community," N10; National Black Women's Health Project, "Targeted Program Development."

62 Cassandra Spratling, "Easy-to-Read, Sister-Sister Style: Health Concerns Facing Black Women," *Boca-Raton News*, April 16, 1995, https://news.google.com /newspapers?nid=1290&dat=19950416&id=eCJUAAAAIBAJ&sjid =iooDAAAAIBAJ&pg=5591,191427&hl=en.

63 Villarosa, *Body and Soul*, back cover.

64 *Essence* is a monthly magazine whose target audience is African American women ages eighteen to forty-nine.

65 Linda Villarosa, "Body and Soul," *Women's Review of Books*, July 1994, 13–14.

66 Cynthia M. Dagnal-Myron, "Book Reaches beyond Basics," *Arizona Daily Star*, January 6, 1995, 1D; Miki Turner, "Guide to Health Focuses Uniquely on Black Women," *Orange County Register*, January 15, 1995, F23.

67 Villarosa, *Body and Soul*, xiv.

68 Spratling, "Easy-to-Read, Sister-Sister Style."

69 Villarosa, "Body and Soul," 13–14.

70 Turner, "Guide to Health Focuses Uniquely on Black Women," F23.

71 Silliman et al., *Undivided Rights*, 71.

72 Ross interview, 2004–2005, 210.

73 Ross interview, 208–209. According to Ross, around the time the NBWHP began writing the self-help manual, tensions between Avery and Allen began to boil over. Ross suggested that Allen feared that her role in the Project would be reduced if they made the self-help process so widely accessible by disseminating the manual. Ross also suggested that the major problem was simply a feeling of competition between Allen and Avery.

74 Byllye Avery, interview by Hannah Dudley-Shotwell, November 2, 2015.

75 Ross interview, 2004–2005, 222.

76 Ross interview, 222; Silliman et al., *Undivided Rights*, 73.

77 Trademark information for Black and Female: What Is the Reality?, http://www

.trademarkia.com/Black-and-female-what-is-the-reality-73735692.html; Ross interview, 2004–2005, 210–211; Be Present, Inc., Black & Female Leadership Training Retreat Workshop, http://www.bepresent.org/images/stories/2015-06-11 _B&F_June_2015_FINAL.pdf.

78 Ross interview, 2004–2005, 210–211. The conflict grew increasingly ugly. Many NBWHP employees felt that they had to take sides. Ross recalls that she had a terrible time deciding what to do, because she felt loyal to Avery but also really devoted to the self-help process.

79 Silliman et al., *Undivided Rights*, 76. The supporters had physical fights. Once, a woman even brought a gun to work and put it on her desk "just to let people know not to fuck with her." Ross interview, 2004–2005, 210–211.

80 Silliman et al., *Undivided Rights*, 76.

81 Ross interview, 2004–2005, 220–221.

82 Silliman et al., *Undivided Rights*, 80–81.

83 Dazon Dixon Diallo, Voices of Feminism Oral History Project, interview by Loretta Ross, April 4, 2009, 4–5.

84 HIV is short for human immunodeficiency virus. It attacks white blood cells and makes it hard for the body to fight infection. AIDS is short for acquired immuno-deficiency syndrome and can develop as a result of HIV, especially if an infected person does not receive treatment.

85 HIV/AIDS Epidemic, Georgetown Law, http://guides.ll.georgetown.edu/c.php?g =592919&p=4182199; A Timeline of HIV and AIDS, HIV.gov, https://www.hiv .gov/hiv-basics/overview/history/hiv-and-aids-timeline.

86 Lawrence K. Altman, "New Homosexual Disorder Worries Health Officials," *New York Times*, May 11, 1982, https://www.nytimes.com/1982/05/11/science/new -homosexual-disorder-worries-health-officials.html?pagewanted=all.

87 HIV/AIDS Epidemic; A Timeline of HIV and AIDS.

88 Altman, "New Homosexual Disorder Worries Health Officials."

89 "History of HIV and AIDS Overview," Avert, https://www.avert.org /professionals/history-hiv-aids/overview.

90 Stina Stoderling and Alison Bernstein, "Dazon Dixon Diallo: Feminism and the Fight to Combat HIV/AIDS," in *Junctures in Women's Leadership: Social Movements*, ed. Mary Trigg and Alison Bernstein (New Brunswick, NJ: Rutgers University Press, 2016).

91 "History of HIV and AIDS Overview.

92 Stoderling and Bernstein, "Dazon Dixon Diallo."

93 AID Atlanta/SisterLove, "Needs Assessment draft," box 35, folder 2: "SisterLove, 1990–94," Ross Papers, SSC.

94 Stoderling and Bernstein, "Dazon Dixon Diallo."

95 Nelson, *More Than Medicine*, 158–162; Dixon Diallo interview, 2009.

96 Stoderling and Bernstein, "Dazon Dixon Diallo."

97 Dixon Diallo interview, 2009, 7.

98 Stoderling and Bernstein, "Dazon Dixon Diallo"; "The Rise of SisterLove during the Stigma of HIV/AIDs," YouTube video, 4:56, posted by Ms. Magazine, September 16, 2016, https://www.youtube.com/watch?v=bm8c14B6SdU.

99 Stoderling and Bernstein, "Dazon Dixon Diallo." The FWHC shifted the clinic's focus away from some of their efforts to address HIV/AIDS but kept open an AIDS hotline. Women's health movement historian Jennifer Nelson argues in *More Than Medicine* that this hotline and the continued relationship between the

FWHC and SisterLove "demonstrated that women of color had impacted the women's health movement so that it better served their interests" (166).

100 Stoderling and Bernstein, "Dazon Dixon Diallo."

101 AID Atlanta/SisterLove, Needs Assessment draft.

102 Shelia Poole, "SisterLove Marks 20 Years," *Atlanta Journal-Constitution*, July 25, 2009, 2B.

103 Jan Gehorsam, "AIDS Harder on Blacks Because of Poverty," *Atlanta Journal-Constitution*, March 8, 1992, D8.

104 Quoted in Poole, "SisterLove Marks 20 Years." The U.S. government was essentially silent about women's ability to contract HIV/AIDS until the CDC acknowledged it in 1993.

105 Stoderling and Bernstein, "Dazon Dixon Diallo."

106 Stoderling and Bernstein.

107 Stoderling and Bernstein.

108 AID Atlanta/SisterLove, Needs Assessment draft.

109 Kenneth Rollins, "Doing CPR on SisterLove: The Founder of the AIDS Program Returns to Save It from Financial Failure," *Atlanta Journal-Constitution*, August 14, 1997, 10D; SisterLove, Inc., "Program/Service Update," *Lovenotes* 2:4 (Fall 1995), box 35, folder 2: "SisterLove, 1990–94," Ross Papers, SSC.

110 SisterLove, Inc., "Love House Program Description," box 35, folder 2: "SisterLove, 1990–94," Ross Papers, SSC.

111 Dixon Diallo interview, 2009, 9.

112 Dixon Diallo interview, 2009, 26–27.

113 Ross interview, 2015.

114 Charon Asetoyer, interview by Justina Licata and Hannah Dudley-Shotwell, September 29, 2017; Charon Asetoyer, Voices of Feminism Oral History Project, interview by Joyce Follet, September 1–2, 2005.

115 Centers for Disease Control and Prevention, National Center for Health Statistics, "Infant Mortality Rates, by race: United States, selected years, 1950–2015," accessed August 8, 2019, available https://www.cdc.gov/nchs/data/hus/2016/011.pdf; "The Socioeconomic, Health and Reproductive Status of Native American Women," May 10, 1990, box 18, folder 9: "Native Women's Reproductive Rights Coalition Conferences, Empowerment through Dialogue, 16–18 May 1990," NAWHERCR, SSC. See also Jeffrey Ian Ross, *American Indians at Risk* (Santa Barbara, CA: ABC-CLIO, 2014).

116 Rife and Dellapenna, *Caring and Curing*.

117 Gurr, *Reproductive Justice*.

118 Charon Asetoyer, interview by Larry Greenfield, September 29, 1997; Gurr, *Reproductive Justice*.

119 Asetoyer interview, 2018.

120 Asetoyer, Cronk, and Hewakapuge, *Indigenous Women's Health Book*, 5.

121 Asetoyer interview, 2005, 22; Native American Women's Health Education Resource Center, accessed April 4, 2014, http://www.nativeshop.org/. The other founders were Clarence Rockboy, Everdale Song Hawk, Jackie Rouse, and Lorenzo Dion. The founders all lived on or near the Yankton Sioux Reservation.

122 Sara M., "Heroes and Heroines," *Mother Jones*, January 1990, box 1, folder 2: "News Clippings, 1988–1991, n.d.," NAWHERCR, SSC. Native American men and women had rates of alcoholism higher than any other ethnic group in the United States. See Silliman et al., *Undivided Rights*, 145–147; M. Annette Jaimes,

The State of Native America: Genocide, Colonization, and Resistance (Boston: South End Press, 1992).

123 Asetoyer interview, 2005, 28; Asetoyer, Cronk, and Hewakapuge, *Indigenous Women's Health Book*, 108; Charon Asetoyer, "Native American Health Center," *Morena Women's Press*, May 1988, box 1, folder 2: "News Clippings, 1988–1991, n.d.," NAWHERCR, SSC; Sue Ivey, "Center Gives Women, Children Health Aid," *Yankton Daily Press*, May 18, 1988, box 1, folder 2: "News Clippings, 1988–1991, n.d.," NAWHERCR, SSC.

124 Asetoyer interview, 2005, 28–34; W. Kline, *Bodies of Knowledge*; Asetoyer interview, 2018; Native American Community Board, "Native American Women's Health Education Resource Center," box 19, folder 2: "Brochures and Fact Sheets, General, n.d.," NAWHERCR, SSC.

125 Asetoyer wrote a proposal for a "Women and Children and Alcohol" program for the NACB and operated it briefly out of her basement.

126 Quoted in Sara M., "Heroes and Heroines."

127 Asetoyer interview, 2005, 28.

128 Hart, "Building a More Inclusive Women's Health Movement," 200.

129 The NLHO was a self-help-based organization for Latina women that also began in the 1980s. They used a version of psychological self-help that was very similar to the NBWHP's to address community concerns such as violence. There is little published literature on their use of self-help to date.

130 Native American Community Board, "Native American Women's Health Education Resource Center," *Wicozanni Wowapi: Good Health Newsletter*, Spring/Summer 1988, box 19, folder 25: "*Wicozanni Wowapi Good Health Newsletter*," NAWHERCR, SSC.

131 Hart, "Building a More Inclusive Movement," 205.

132 NAWHERC works on local, regional, national, and international levels. In addition to the direct services on the Yankton Sioux Reservation, it also gathers information and provides referrals for indigenous women who live in an area the Bureau of Indian Affairs defines as the "Aberdeen" or "Plains" area (North Dakota, South Dakota, Iowa, and Nebraska). Meanwhile, its leaders often participate in national and international efforts to improve the overall health of indigenous women. See Silliman et al., *Undivided Rights*, 144; Sara M., "Heroes and Heroines."

133 Silliman et al., *Undivided Rights*, 145.

134 Asetoyer interview, 2018.

135 Asetoyer interview, 2018.

136 Asetoyer believed the process did not go far enough to promote healing. "It's like opening up that Pandora's box and letting the floodgate open," she said. She saw the NBWHP's psychological self-help as "kind of like a band-aid" that just hid a wound and did not encourage it to heal. Asetoyer interview, 2005.

137 Asetoyer interview, 2005; Silliman et al., *Undivided Rights*, 148–149.

138 Silliman et al., *Undivided Rights*, 148.

139 NAWHERC reports that they have influenced changes to federal policies around issues such as informed consent and patient confidentiality. Silliman et al., *Undivided Rights*, 150–151; NAWHERC, "Indigenous Women's Dialogue: Roundtable Report on the Accessibility of Plan B as an Over the Counter (OTC) within Indian Health Service," February 2012, http://www.nativeshop.org/images /stories/media/pdfs/Plan-B-Report.pdf.

140 Native American Community Board, "Native American Women's Health
     Education Resource Center," box 1, folder 1: "General, 1988–2006, n.d.,"
     NAWHERCR, SSC; NAWHERC, "Administrative Associate," box 3, folder 16:
     "Job Descriptions, 1993, n.d.," NAWHERCR, SSC.

141 Asetoyer interview, 2005, 39.

142 NAWHERC also developed literature on a variety of other issues. In 1988,
     NAWHERC began developing "culturally specific materials" to address nutrition.
     Because poverty is so pervasive on reservations, Native Americans often had very
     poor diets. They hoped to encourage participants to learn about nutrition and
     about the effects of poor nutrition so that they could take an active role in
     preventing conditions such as diabetes and high blood pressure. Their literature
     highlighted foods that Native Americans would have included in their diet before
     European colonization. Silliman et al., *Undivided Rights*, 153; Native American
     Community Board, press release, box 1, folder 1: "General, 1988–2006, n.d.,"
     NAWHERCR, SSC; Asetoyer, Cronk, and Hewakapuge, *Indigenous Women's
     Health Book*, 177.

143 Native American Community Board, "Native American Women's Health
     Education Resource Center," box 19, folder 2: "Brochures and Fact Sheets,
     General, n.d.," NAWHERCR, SSC.

144 Asetoyer interview, 2005, 57; Donna Haukaas "Empowerment through Dialogue:
     Native American Women Hold Historic Meeting," box 18, folder 9: "Native
     Women's Reproductive Rights Coalition Conferences, Empowerment through
     Dialogue, 16–18 May 1990," NAWHERCR, SSC.

145 Sonya Shin and Charon Asetoyer, "The Positive Impact of Community Based
     Self-Help Education among the Native American Diabetic Population of the
     Yankton Sioux Reservation," 1991, box 14, folder 10: "'The Positive Impact of
     Community Based Self-Help Education . . .' by Sonya Shin and Charon Asetoyer,
     1991," NAWHERCR, SSC; Asetoyer interview, 2018. NAWHERC staff saw that
     many women who abused alcohol or had partners who abused alcohol were in
     violent relationships. They believed that in order to help themselves, these women
     would have to remove themselves from such relationships. In 1991, NAWHERC
     opened the Women's Lodge, a shelter to house Native women and children who
     were survivors of domestic violence and to help the women find jobs, medical
     referrals, and support groups. Native American Community Board, "Services,"
     accessed December 1, 2015, http://nativeshop.org/programs-and-services
     .html#shelter.

146 Dixon Diallo interview, 2009, 51–52.

Notes to Chapter 6

Epigraph: "After *Roe v. Wade*," clippings from Rebecca Chalker's personal papers.

1 Murphy, "Immodest Witnessing: The Epistemology of Vaginal Self-Examination
   in the U.S. Feminist Self-Help Movement." *Feminist Studies* 30 (2004): 115–147;
   W. Kline, *Bodies of Knowledge: Sexuality, Reproduction, and Women's Health in
   the Second Wave* (Chicago: University of Chicago Press, 2010); Morgen, *Into Our
   Own Hands: The Women's Health Movement in the United States, 1969–1990* (New
   Brunswick, NJ: Rutgers University Press, 2002).

2 Denise Copelton, a scholar of sociology, has written the most extensive

exploration of post-*Roe* menstrual extraction to date. She argues that feminist self-help persists even today, including in the form of menstrual extraction, and closely examines a twentieth-century self-help group. See Copelton, "Menstrual Extraction, Abortion, and the Political Context of Feminist Self-Help," *Advances in Gender Research* 8 (2004): 129–164.

3 Gilmore, *Groundswell: Grassroots Feminist Activism in Postwar America* (New York: Routledge, Taylor and Francis Group, 2013).

4 Gilmore, 158.

5 "Self-Abortion Controversy," *Mother Jones*, April 1981, 8. The Federation of Feminist Women's Health Centers acquired an automatic typesetter, and volunteers from the clinics typeset the book themselves. Personal correspondence with Carol Downer, January 5, 2016.

6 Quoted in Eberhardt Press, "Free to Choose."

7 "Self-Abortion Controversy," 8.

8 Erika Thorne, "Sustaining the Women's Self-Help Movement," *EqualTime*, May 23–June 6, 1990, 9, box 56, folder: "ME Articles," FWHCR, SBC.

9 Celine, "Failed Abortion Book," *off our backs*, August–September 1980, 25.

10 Mecca Rylance and Tacie Dejanikus, "Pro & Anti-choice Dialogue: Cooptation or Cooperation," *off our backs*, March 31, 1979, 4–5, 28.

11 Suzann Gage, "Speculum Press[es] Points," *off our backs*, August-September 1980, 24.

12 Italics in original. The two reviewers were Catherine Edwards and Alison Stirling. Edwards was a member of a collective that produced the feminist journal *Hysteria*, and Stirling worked for Planned Parenthood. Edwards and Stirling, "Reviews: When Birth Control Fails . . . How to Abort Ourselves Safely," *Healthsharing: A Canadian Women's Health Quarterly* 2:1 (Winter 1980): 22, http://www.cwhn .ca/sites/default/files/PDF/Healthsharing/1980_Healthsharing_Vol_2_No_1 _Winter.pdf.

13 Celine, "Failed Abortion Book," 25.

14 Violent incidents aimed at abortion providers were few and far between in the years immediately following *Roe*. See Joffe, *Dispatches from the Abortion Wars: The Costs of Fanaticism to Doctors, Patients, and the Rest of Us* (Boston: Beacon Press, 2009), 49; Joffe, *Doctors of Conscience: The Struggle to Provide Abortion before and after Roe v. Wade* (Boston: Beacon Press, 1995), 5. The National Abortion Federation (NAF) did not begin tracking incidents of violence and disruption at clinics until 1977. NAF reported 149 total incidents of violence and disruption against abortion and of disruption against abortion providers from 1977 to 1983. (Figures were not available for individual years.) In 1984, they reported 131 incidents. In 1985, they reported 149, and in 1986, 133. These were the peak years, and nothing higher than 72 was reported after that for the remainder of the 1980s. Picketing and harassment continued, however, especially after Operation Rescue was founded. See National Abortion Federation to NAF Affiliates, "Incidents of Violence and Disruption against Abortion Providers," box 56, folder: "Clinic Violence—NAF (1990)," FWHCR, SBC; "Violence against U.S. Abortion Clinics Intensifies," National Abortion Federation press release, September 14, 1990, box 56, folder: "Clinic Violence—NAF (1990)," FWHCR, SBC.

15 Nelson, *More Than Medicine: A History of the Feminist Women's Health Movement* (New York: New York University Press, 2015), 146–148.

16 Lynne Randall, "Executive Director's Report for 1985," box 7, folder: "Administrative Files General, FWHC Executive Summary," FWHCR, SBC.

17 Randall.

18 Nelson, *More Than Medicine*, 148–149.

19 "Sequence of Anti-Abortion Activity, Feminist Women's Health Center, Atlanta, Georgia," July 19, 1985– January 12, 1986, box 52, folder: "Anti Activity Chronology 1985," FWHCR, SBC.

20 Jan Gehorsam, "In the Hands of Women," *Atlanta Journal-Constitution*, January 7, 1992, D1. Operation Rescue, founded in the mid-1980s by Randall Terry, was an extremist group of protesters who targeted clinics, as well as abortion providers and their families. Today, this group has splintered into those who follow Terry and those who disapprove of his tactics, instead following the group's new leader, Troy Newman. See Operation Rescue, accessed June 3, 2012, http://www.operationrescue.org/about-us/history/.

21 Rose, *Safe, Legal, and Unavailable? Abortion Politics in the United States* (Washington, DC: CQ Press, 2007), 109–110.

22 *Webster vs. Reproductive Health Services*, 492 U.S. 490 (1989), U.S. Supreme Court, Find Law, accessed March 22, 2012, http://laws.findlaw.com/us/492/490.html; *Roe v. Wade*, Legal Information Institute, accessed March 21, 2012, http://www.law.cornell.edu/supct/html/historics/USSC_CR_0410_0113_ZS.html.

23 "Self Help Abortion Video Fights Back," *Feminist Women's Health Center Newsletter*, Spring 1990, box 57, folder: "Newsletter–Spring 1990," FWHCR, SBC.

24 Federation of Feminist Women's Health Centers, "Protect Your Right to a Safe Abortion—Support the 1990 Self-Help Tour," flyer, box 61, folder: "SH Tour," FWHCR, SBC.

25 Carol Downer to Pro-choice Supporters [who ordered *No Going Back*], box 61, folder: "SH Tour," FWHCR, SBC.

26 Federation of Feminist Women's Health Centers, *No Going Back: A Pro-choice Perspective*, VHS, directed by Carol Downer (Los Angeles, CA, 1989).

27 Cynthia Gorney, "The Grandmother and the Abortion Kit: On the Feminist Fringe, an Alarming Tactic," *Washington Post*, October 4, 1989, box 56, folder: "ME Articles," FWHCR, SBC.

28 Karen Tumulty, "Alternative to Clinics: Feminists Teaching Home Procedure," *Los Angeles Times*, August 14, 1989, copy in box 62, folder: "ME Coverage (3 of 4)," FWHCR, SBC.

29 L. K. Brown to M. E. Tour Planning Group / Federation of FWHCs, December 4, 1989, box 61, folder: "SH Tour," FWHCR, SBC.

30 L. K. Brown to M. E. Tour Planning Group; Morgen, *Into Our Own Hands*, 103; L. K. Brown to FFWHC Press Committee, November 10, 1989, box 61, folder: "SH Tour," FWHCR, SBC.

31 "Menstrual Extraction: Is It Another Question of Choice?," *Dallas Morning News*, July 20, 1989, 12C, copy in box 62, folder: "ME Coverage (3 of 4)," FWHCR, SBC.

32 Kim Painter and Dennis Kelly, "Calling a Halt to Home Abortion Kits," *USA Today*, August 15, 1989, 1D.

33 Carol Downer to Richard Steele, Harry and Grace Steele Foundation, box 61, folder: "SH Tour," FWHCR, SBC; Deborah Fleming and Janet Callum, "Self Help / ME Tour Midwest," April 21–29, 1990," box 61, folder: "Tour (ME)," FWHCR, SBC.

34 Rina Berkhout to Ami Hofwomy and Chris Marzicano, April 4, 1990, box 61, folder: "SH Tour," FWHCR, SBC.

35 Fleming and Callum, "Self Help / ME Tour Midwest."

36 Jodi Duckett, "At Home Abortion High Risk—Women Unite to Sidestep Restrictions," *Times Union* (Albany), August 18, 1992, C1.

37 In one memo, a member of the tour planning committee noted that some of their contacts may have described themselves as poor, but the committee did not see them that way. L. K. Brown to M. E. Tour Planning Group / Federation of FWHCs.

38 "Refuse and Resist," last modified September 17, 2008, accessed June 3, 2012, http://www.refuseandresist.org/.

39 Fleming and Callum, "Self Help / ME Tour Midwest."

40 Fleming and Callum.

41 Downer to Pro-choice Supporters, FWHCR, SBC.

42 Quoted in Gorney, "The Grandmother and the Abortion Kit."

43 Gehorsam, "In the Hands of Women," D1; "Women Turn to Self-Help Groups for Abortions, Despite the Risks," *New York Times*, September 9, 1992, C13.

44 Jill Benderly, "New Videos on Abortion, Breast Cancer, Menopause," *New Directions for Women*, July/August 1989, box 56, folder: "ME Articles," FWHCR, SBC.

45 Tensions between physicians and "irregular" medical practitioners, especially midwives, date back to the nineteenth century. Fearful of competition from outside their ranks, the American Medical Association (AMA) pushed to make abortion illegal in order to establish state control over the procedure. By 1880, most states in the United States had criminalized abortion, with the exception of "therapeutic abortion" in the event that a birth threatened a woman's life. This gave physicians even more control, allowing them, but not a pregnant woman, to decide when an abortion might be necessary. Reagan, *When Abortion Was a Crime: Women, Medicine, and the Law in the United States, 1867–1973* (Berkeley: University of California Press, 1998); W. Kline, *Bodies of Knowledge*; personal correspondence with Rebecca Chalker on August 13, 2015.

46 "National Abortion Federation," accessed March 22, 2012, http://www.prochoice.org/about_naf/index.html; Duckett, "At Home Abortion High Risk," C1.

47 Gehorsam, "In the Hands of Women," D1.

48 Mimi Hall, "Some Groups Teaching Do-It-Yourself Abortions," *USA Today*, January 29, 1992, 5A.

49 Hall; Rios, "Abortions at Home"; "Some Women Are Teaching Each Other How to Perform Early-Term Abortions," *San Antonio Express-News*, August 31, 1991, 17A.

50 Charles Truehart, "Clash Looms over At Home Abortion," *Washington Post*, October 22, 1991, C7.

51 Rothman, "Menstrual Extraction."

52 Truehart, "Clash Looms over At Home Abortion," C7.

53 Gehorsam, "In the Hands of Women," D1; Truehart, "Clash Looms over At Home Abortion," C7.

54 Elaine Herscher, "Women Seek Abortion Know-How/Preparing for Overturning of Roe vs. Wade," *San Francisco Chronicle*, June 28, 1991, A1.

55 Before being banned, the Del-Em was widely available because of its price (at $89.95, it was more affordable than many forms of abortion), and after the ban,

women could still put them together relatively cheaply on their own with the instructions the Federation made available. Instructions were available in Gage, *When Birth Control Fails: How to Abort Ourselves Safely* (Hollywood, CA: Speculum Press, 1979).

56 John McGuire, "Groups Not Seen Here Yet," *St. Louis Post-Dispatch*, February 6, 1992, 1E.

57 Gehorsam, "In the Hands of Women," D1; Rose, *Safe, Legal, and Unavailable?*, 90.

58 Because of their own limited resources, the Federation often focused on media attention for menstrual extraction instead of teaching the procedure directly to low-income or rural women.

59 Leigh Fenly, "Abortion Kit Earns Friends, Enemies," *San Diego Union*, August 21, 1989, D1; Jan Gehorsham, "Legal Climate Spurs Home Abortion Advocates," *St. Louis Post-Dispatch*, February 6, 1992, 1E; Silliman et al., *Undivided Rights*, 63.

60 Fenly, "Abortion Kit Earns Friends, Enemies," D1; Gehorsham, "Legal Climate Spurs Home Abortion Advocates," 1E.

61 Ellen Bilofsky, "After *Webster* . . . If Abortion Becomes Illegal," *Health/PAC Bulletin*, Winter 1989, 24–26.

62 Reagan, *When Abortion Was a Crime*, 210–215.

63 Bilofsky, "After *Webster* . . . If Abortion Becomes Illegal," 24–26.

64 Tanfer Emin Tunc, "Innovators and Instigators: Feminist Contributions to American Abortion Technology, 1963–1973," *Journal of Family Planning and Reproductive Healthcare* 33:3 (August 2007): 149–154.

65 Quoted in Gehorsham, "Legal Climate Spurs Home Abortion Advocates," 1E.

66 "The Art of Giving When Your Resources Are Vast," *Bloomberg Business*, October 24, 1999, accessed January 16, 2016, http://www.bloomberg.com/bw /stories/1999-10-24/the-art-of-giving-when-your-resources-are-vast.

67 Painter and Kelly, "Calling a Halt to Home Abortion Kits," 1D.

68 "Health Care Activists to Teach Do-It-Yourself Abortions," *Sun-Sentinel*, July 30, 1989, 13A, box 62, folder: "ME Coverage (3 of 4)," FWHCR, SBC; Tour Contacts, box 61, folder: "SH Tour," FWHCR, SBC.

69 "Home Abortion Kit Making the Rounds," *Worcester Telegram and Gazette*, July 30, 1989, A10; Downer and Chalker, *A Woman's Book of Choices*, 117; Donna Vavala, "Home Abortions on NOW Agenda," *Tampa Tribune*, October 8, 1991, 1; "U. Professor to Lecture on Home Abortion," *Salt Lake Tribune*, January 7, 1992, D2; Gehorsham, "Legal Climate Spurs Home Abortion Advocates," 1E; Nancy Hobbs, "Utah Women Learn How to Do Home Abortion," *Salt Lake Tribune*, January 11, 1992, A1.

70 "Home Abortion Kit Making the Rounds," A10.

71 Gilmore, *Groundswell*.

72 Vavala, "Home Abortions on NOW Agenda," 1.

73 Anastasia Toufexis, "Abortions without Doctors," *Time*, August 28, 1989, box 62, folder: "ME Coverage (2 of 4)," FWHCR, SBC. Ireland later became the president of NOW from 1991 to 2001. See "Patricia Ireland, Former President, 1991–2001," National Organization for Women, accessed June 2, 2012, http:// www.now.org/officers/pi.html.

74 Quoted in Hall, "Some Groups Teaching Do-It-Yourself Abortions," 5A.

75 Quoted in "U. Professor to Lecture on Home Abortion," D2.

76 *Planned Parenthood of Southeastern Pa. v. Casey*, Legal Information Institute,

accessed March 21, 2012, http://www.law.cornell.edu/supct/html/91-744.ZS
.html.

77 Today, many view *Casey* as a precursor to Targeted Regulation of Abortion
Provider (TRAP) laws, regulations that place burdens on abortion providers but
not other medical officials. See NARAL, "Targeted Regulation of Abortion
Providers (TRAP)," accessed January 13, 2016, http://www.prochoiceamerica.org
/what-is-choice/fast-facts/issues-trap.html; Guttmacher Institute, "State Policies
in Brief: "Targeted Regulation of Abortion Providers," January 1, 2016, accessed
January 13, 2016, http://www.guttmacher.org/statecenter/spibs/spib_TRAP.pdfl;
"Home Abortion to Be Topic," *Sun-Sentinel*, July 22, 1992, 3B.

Notes to Epilogue

1 Though many believe that it is an abbreviation of "magazine," the word "zine" is
short for "fanzine," a term that dates to the 1930s, when science-fiction fans began
self-publishing stories and trading them with each other. Alison Piepmeier, *Girl
Zines: Making Media, Doing Feminism* (New York: New York University Press,
2009), xii.

2 Piepmeier, 4.

3 Cindy, *Doris*, no. 15, Niku Arbabi Zine Collection, SBC. Most zines did not
include a publication date.

4 *Oompa! Oompa!*, Sarah Wood Zine Collection, SBC.

5 Kate Eichhorn, *The Archival Turn in Feminism: Outrage in Order* (Philadelphia:
Temple University Press, 2013), 70.

6 Piepmeier, *Girl Zines*.

7 For example, *Our Bodies, Ourselves* based each of its new editions on changes
suggested by readers, and in-person self-help groups always emphasized dialogue
and the importance of group knowledge production. See W. Kline, "'Please
Include This in Your Book': Readers Respond to Our Bodies, Ourselves," *Bulletin
of the History of Medicine* 79:1 (2005): 81–110.

8 Susannah Fox and Maeve Duggan, "Health Online 2013," Pew Research Center's
Internet and American Life Project, January 15, 2013, accessed December 14, 2015,
http://www.pewinternet.org/files/old-media//Files/Reports/PIP_HealthOnline
.pdf.

9 The Beautiful Cervix Project, accessed December 4, 2015, http://www
.beautifulcervix.com/.

10 There are many examples of such online communities. See, for example, Daily
Strength, "Trying to Conceive Support Group," accessed August 8, 2019,
http://www.dailystrength.org/c/Trying-To-Conceive/support-group; Baby
Center, accessed August 8, 2019, http://community.babycenter.com/groups/topic
/2/getting_pregnant; Momtastic, "Baby and Bump," accessed August 8, 2019,
http://babyandbump.momtastic.com; Two Week Wait, accessed August 8, 2019,
http://www.twoweekwait.com/community/.

11 See Northwest Cryobank, "Trying to Conceive," accessed August 8, 2019,
http://www.iamtryingtoconceive.com; Essential Baby, "Assisted Conception,"
accessed August 8, 2019, http://www.essentialbaby.com.au/forums/index.php?
/forum/37-assisted-conception-general.

12 Susan Gerber, "The Evolving Gender Gap in General Obstetrics," *American
Journal of Obstetrics and Gynecology* 195, no. 5 (2006): 1427–1430.

13 Morgen, *Into Our Own Hands: The Women's Health Movement in the United States, 1969–1990* (New Brunswick, NJ: Rutgers University Press, 2002), 149.

14 See, for example, GW Center for Integrative Medicine, accessed January 10, 2016, http://www.gwcim.com/services/womens-health-and-holistic-gynecology/.

15 On the depoliticization of feminism in both health and other arenas, see Kristin J. Anderson, *Modern Misogyny: Anti-Feminism in a Post-Feminist Era* (New York: Oxford University Press, 2014); Dorothy E. Chunn, Susan Boyd, and Hester Lessard, *Reaction and Resistance: Feminism, Law, and Social Change* (Vancouver, BC: UBC Press, 2007); Jo Reger, *Everywhere and Nowhere: Contemporary Feminism in the United States* (New York: Oxford University Press, 2012); Morgen, *Into Our Own Hands*.

16 NAWHERC, "Dakota Talk Radio," accessed March 11, 2019, http://nativeshop .org/programs/dakota-talk-radio.html.

17 Be Present, Inc., "Black and Female Leadership Initiative Participants," accessed March 11, 2019, http://bepresent.org/images/Be%20Present_Black%20&%20 Female%20Institute_Select%20Bios_FINAL.pdf.

18 Be Present, Inc., "Our Story, Mission, Vision, and Core Values," accessed March 11, 2019, http://www.bepresent.org/history.html; Be Present, Inc., "Black and Female Leadership Initiative Participants."

19 "The Herstory of SisterSong," 2003, box 5, folder: "Meetings: National Conference Training I," Luz Marina Rodriquez Papers, SSC.

20 The group began with sixteen founding organizations, and by the twenty-first century, there were approximately eighty affiliate groups. SisterSong, *Collective Voices*, November 13, 2003, box 11, folder 3: "SisterSong Women of Color Reproductive Health Collective, National Conference, 2003," NAWHERCR, SSC.

21 Feminist Women's Health Center / Cedar River Clinics, accessed December 4, 2015, http://www.fwhc.org/welcome.htm.

22 See Progressive Health Services, "Women's Health—Ob/Gyn," accessed January 10, 2016, http://www.progressivehealth.org/womens-health/.

23 Feminist Women's Health Center, "History," accessed March 11, 2019, https:// www.feministcenter.org/history/.

24 "Shodhini" is a Sanskrit word for female researcher. This group takes its name from a group of women in India who wrote a book titled *Touch Me, Touch Me Not: Women, Plants, and Healing* (New Delhi: Kali for Women, 1997).

25 Shodhini Institute, accessed March 11, 2019, https://shodhiniinstitute.weebly.com/.

26 Shodhini Blogspot, "About Us," accessed December 8, 2015, http://shodhini .blogspot.com.

27 Carol Downer, "Another Second-Wave Feminist Refuses to Be Silenced by Transgender Critics," October 28, 2015, http://femwords.blogspot.com/2015/10 /another-second-wave-feminist-refuses-to.html.

28 "Political Beliefs of the Feminist Women's Health Center," 1976, box 62, folder: "Participatory Clinic," FWHCR, SBC.

Bibliography

Manuscript and Archival Collections

Iowa Women's Archives, University of Iowa Archives, University of Iowa Libraries, Iowa City, Iowa
   Carol Hodne Records
   Emma Goldman Clinic for Women (Iowa City) Records
Sallie Bingham Center for Women's History and Culture, Rubenstein Rare Book and Manuscript Library, Duke University Archives, Durham, North Carolina
   Feminist Women's Health Center Records
   Lesbian Health Resource Center
   Niku Arbabi Zine Collection
   Sarah Dyer Zine Collection
   Sarah Wood Zine Collection
Schlesinger Library, Radcliffe Institute, Harvard University, Cambridge, Massachusetts
   Barbara Seaman Papers
   Boston Women's Health Book Collective, Additional Records
   Boston Women's Health Book Collective Records
   Records of the Mautner Project
   Toni Carabillo and Judith Meuli Papers
   Women's Community Health Center Records
   Women's Newsletter and Periodical Collection
Sophia Smith Collection, Smith College, Northampton, Massachusetts
   Black Women's Health Imperative Records
   Charon Asetoyer Papers
   Health Collection
   Loretta Ross Papers
   Luz Alvarez Martinez Papers
   Luz Marina Rodriquez Papers
   National Women's Health Network Records
   Native American Women's Health Education Resource Center Records
   SisterSong Women of Color Reproductive Justice Collective Records

Walter P. Reuther Library Archives of Labor and Urban Affairs, Wayne State University, Detroit, Michigan
Detroit Feminist Women's Health Center Records

Newspapers and Periodicals

Arizona Star
Atlanta Constitution
Atlanta Journal
Atlanta Journal-Constitution
Atlantic
Boca-Raton News
Cincinnati Post
Dallas Morning News
Deseret News
Gainesville Sun
Gazette (Cedar Rapids-Iowa City)
Health/PAC Bulletin
Healthsharing: A Canadian Women's Health Quarterly
Los Angeles Sentinel
Los Angeles Times
Morning Call
Mother Jones
Ms. Magazine
New Yorker

New York Times
New York Times Magazine
off our backs
On the Issues Magazine
Orange County Register
Publishers Weekly
Quest: A Feminist Quarterly
Ramparts
Salt Lake Tribune
San Antonio Express-News
San Diego Union
Seattle Post-Intelligencer
St. Louis Post-Dispatch
Sun-Sentinel (Broward County)
Tampa Tribune
Times Union (Albany)
USA Today
Washington Post
Women's Review of Books
Worcester Telegram and Gazette

Books (Primary)

Asetoyer, Charon, Katharine Cronk, and Samanthi Hewakapuge. *Indigenous Women's Health Book, within the Sacred Circle: Reproductive Rights, Environmental Health, Traditional Herbs and Remedies.* Lake Andes, SD: Pine Hill Press, 2003.

Cassidy-Brinn, Ginny, Francie Hornstein, and Carol Downer. *Woman-Centered Pregnancy and Birth.* Pittsburgh: Cleis Press, 1984.

Chalker, Rebecca. *The Complete Cervical Cap Guide.* New York: Harper and Row, 1987.

Chaney, Betty Norwood. "Black Women's Health Conference." *Southern Changes* 5 (1983): 18–20.

Corea, Gena. *The Hidden Malpractice: How American Medicine Mistreats Women.* New York: Jove/HBJ, 1977.

Downer, Carol, and Rebecca Chalker. *A Woman's Book of Choices: Abortion, Menstrual Extraction, RU-486.* New York: Seven Stories Press, 1992.

Federation of Feminist Women's Health Centers. *How to Stay Out of the Gynecologist's Office.* Minneapolis: Peace Press, 1981.

———. *A New View of a Woman's Body: A Fully Illustrated Guide.* West Hollywood, CA: Feminist Health Press, 1991.

Frankfort, Ellen. *Vaginal Politics.* New York: Quadrangle Books, 1972.

Gage, Suzann. *When Birth Control Fails: How to Abort Ourselves Safely.* Hollywood, CA: Speculum Press, 1979.

Hepburn, Cuca. *Alive and Well: A Lesbian Health Guide*. Freedom, CA: Crossing Press, 1988.

Hirsch, Lolly. *The Witch's Os*. Stamford, CT: New Moon Publications, 1972.

Lipnack, Jessica, and Jeffrey Stamps. *Networking, the First Report and Directory*. Garden City, NY: Doubleday, 1982.

Reitz, Rosetta. *Menopause: A Positive Approach*. New York: Penguin Books, 1977.

Seaman, Barbara. *Women and the Crisis in Sex Hormones*. New York: Bantam Books, 1977.

Villarosa, Linda. *Body and Soul: The Black Women's Guide to Physical Health and Well-Being*. New York: Harper Perennial, 1994.

Films and Online Videos

Federation of Feminist Women's Health Centers. *No Going Back: A Pro-choice Perspective*. VHS. Directed by Carol Downer. Los Angeles, CA, 1989.

"Origin of the Phrase 'Women of Color.'" YouTube video. Posted by Western States Center, February 15, 2011. https://www.youtube.com/watch?v=82vl34mi4Iw.

"The Rise of SisterLove during the Stigma of HIV/AIDs." YouTube video. Posted by *Ms. Magazine*, September 16, 2016. https://www.youtube.com/watch?v=bm8c14B6SdU.

"Self-Help History / Carol Downer." YouTube video. Posted by Shelby Coleman, November 6, 2014. https://www.youtube.com/watch?v=OqcGfxsLokY.

Women Make Movies. *It's O.K. to Peek: Gynecological Self-Exam; How to Do Self-Exam; What to Look For; When to Seek Medical Assistance*. Directed by S. Pearl Sharp. Los Angeles, CA, 1995.

Oral Histories

AUTHOR'S INTERVIEWS

Asetoyer, Charon. Phone interview (with Justina Licata). September 29, 2017.

Avery, Byllye. Video chat interview. November 2, 2015.

Banzhaf, Marion. Video chat interview. April 24–25, 2015.

Chalker, Rebecca. Video chat Interview. March 19, 2015.

Downer, Carol. Boston, Massachusetts. March 26, 2014.

Downer, Carol. Video chat interview. October 27, 2015.

Hornstein, Francie. Phone interview. June, 2, 2015.

Hornstein, Francie. Interview by Hannah Dudley-Shotwell and Gill Frank for Sexing History. June 1, 2018.

Jimenez, Laura. Phone interview. April 17, 2015.

Peskin, Yael. Interview by Hannah Dudley-Shotwell and Gill Frank for Sexing History. June 25, 2018.

Ross, Loretta. Video chat interview. August 18, 2015.

Smith, Pam. Phone interview. July 26, 2017.

VOICES OF FEMINISM ORAL HISTORY PROJECT INTERVIEWS

Transcripts online at the Sophia Smith Collection website, https://www.smith.edu/library/libs/ssc/vof/vof-intro.html.

Asetoyer, Charon. Interview by Joyce Follet. September 1–2, 2005.

Avery, Byllye. Interview by Loretta Ross. July 21–22, 2005.

Dixon Diallo, Dazon. Interview by Loretta Ross. April 4, 2009.

Martinez, Luz Alvarez. Interview by Loretta Ross. December 6–7, 2004.

Ross, Loretta. Interview by Joyce Follet. November 3–5, 2004; December 1–3, 2004; February 4, 2005.

Other Interviews

Allen, Lillie. Interview by Loretta Ross. Loretta Ross Papers. Smith College. 2003.

Asetoyer, Charon. Interview by Larry Greenfield. Charon Asetoyer Papers. Smith College. September 29, 1997.

Avery, Byllye. Interview by Rose Norman for Sinister Wisdom. February 2013. http://www.sinisterwisdom.org/SW93Supplement/Avery.

Banzhaf, Marion. Interview by Sarah Schulman for ACT UP Oral History Project. April 18, 2007. http://www.actuporalhistory.org/interviews/images/banzhaf.pdf.

Gage, Suzann. Interview by Bonnie Fortune. August 2009. http://www.bonniefortune.info/overview/temporary-conversations-suzann-gage/.

Hasper, Dido. Interview by Gayle Kimball. *Women's Culture: The Women's Resistance of the Seventies*. Metuchen, NJ: Scarecrow Press. 1981.

Smith, Pam. Interview by Barbara Esrig for Sinister Wisdom. Additional edits by Rose Norman. N.D. http://www.sinisterwisdom.org/SW93Supplement/Smith.

Selected Websites

Beautiful Cervix Project. http://www.beautifulcervix.com/.

Black Women's Health Imperative. http://www.Blackwomenshealth.org/.

Feminist Women's Health Center in Atlanta. http://www.feministcenter.org/.

Feminist Women's Health Center in Washington State. http://www.fwhc.org/.

National Institutes of Health. http://www.nlm.nih.gov/.

National Latina Health Organization. http://clnet.ucla.edu/women/nlho/.

National Women's Health Network: A Voice for Women, a Network for Change. https://nwhn.org/.

Native American Women's Health Education Resource Center. http://www.nativeshop.org/.

SisterLove, Inc. http://sisterlove.org/.

SisterSong Women of Color Reproductive Justice. http://www.sistersong.net/index.php.

Women's Health in Women's Hands. http://womenshealthinwomenshands.org/.

Women's Health Specialists. http://www.womenshealthspecialists.org/.

Unpublished Dissertations

Brown, Laura. "Blood Rumors: An Exploration of the Meaning in the Stories of a Contemporary Menstrual Practice." PhD diss., California Institute for Integral Studies, 2002.

Choi, Mihwa. "Contesting *Imaginaires* in Death Rituals during the Northern Song Dynasty." PhD diss., University of Chicago, 2008.

Chuppa-Cornell, Kimberly K. "Days of Silence: A Content Analysis of Women's Health Information in *Good Housekeeping* Magazine, 1920–1965." PhD diss., Arizona State University, 1993.

Dayi, Ayse. "The Empowerment of Women in Reproductive Services: A Poststructural Feminist Case Study of Two Women's Health Centers." PhD diss., Pennsylvania State University, 2005.

Eubank, Christine E. "The Speculum and the Cul-de-Sac: Suburban Feminism in the 1960s and 1970s, Orange County, California." PhD diss., University of California, Irvine, 2013.

Hart, Evan. "Building a More Inclusive Women's Health Movement: Byllye Avery and the Development of the National Black Women's Health Project, 1981–1990." PhD diss., University of Cincinnati, 2012.

Keane, Katarina. "Second-Wave Feminism in the American South, 1965–1980." PhD diss., University of Maryland, College Park, 2009.

MacPherson, Kathleen I. "Feminist Praxis in the Making: The Menopause Collective." PhD diss., Brandeis University, 1986.

Rosenbaum, Judith Aliza Hyman. "Whose Bodies? Whose Selves? A History of American Women's Health Activism, 1968–Present." PhD diss., Brown University, 2004.

Ruzek, Sheryl Kendra. "The Women's Health Movement: Finding Alternatives to Traditional Medical Professionalism." PhD diss., University of California, Davis, 1977.

Books and Articles (Secondary)

Agigian, Amy. *Baby Steps: How Lesbian Alternative Insemination Is Changing the World*. Middletown, CT: Wesleyan University Press, 2004.

Anderson, Kristin J. *Modern Misogyny: Anti-Feminism in a Post-Feminist Era*. New York: Oxford University Press, 2014.

Baehr, Ninia. *Abortion without Apology: A Radical History for the 1990s*. Boston: South End Press, 1990.

Baer, Hans A. *Biomedicine and Alternative Healing Systems in America: Issues of Class, Race, Ethnicity, and Gender*. Madison: University of Wisconsin Press, 2001.

Baird, Karen, Dana-Ain Davis, and Kimberly Christensen. *Beyond Reproduction: Women's Health, Activism, and Public Policy*. Madison, NJ: Fairleigh Dickinson University Press, 2009.

Barnes, Teresa. "Not until Zimbabwe Is Free Can We Stop to Think about It: The Zimbabwe African National Union and Radical Women's Health Activists in the United States, 1979." *Radical History Review* 119 (2014): 53–71.

Bart, Pauline. "Seizing the Means of Reproduction: An Illegal Feminist Abortion Collective—How and Why It Worked." *Qualitative Sociology* 10:4 (1987): 339–357.

Baumgardner, Jennifer. *Abortion and Life*. New York: Akashic Books, 2008.

Baxandall, Rosalyn, and Linda Gordon. Introduction to *Dear Sisters: Dispatches from the Women's Liberation Movement*, edited by Rosalyn Baxandall and Linda Gordon. New York: Basic Books, 2000.

Beito, David T. *From Mutual Aid to the Welfare State: Fraternal Societies and Social Services, 1890–1967*. Chapel Hill: University of North Carolina Press, 2000.

Berkeley, Kathleen. *The Women's Liberation Movement in America*. Westport, CT: Greenwood Press, 1999.

Blackwell, Maylei. *Chicana Power: Contested Histories of Feminism in the Chicana Movement*. Austin: University of Texas Press, 2011.

Bobel, Chris. *New Blood: Third Wave Feminism and the Politics of Menstruation*. New Brunswick, NJ: Rutgers University Press, 2010.

Borkman, Thomasina Jo. *Understanding Self-Help/Mutual Aid: Experiential Learning in the Commons*. New Brunswick, NJ: Rutgers University Press, 1999.

Breines, Wini. *The Trouble between Us: An Uneasy History of White and Black Women in the Feminist Movement*. New York: Oxford University Press, 2006.

Brownmiller, Susan. *In Our Time: Memoir of a Revolution.* New York: Dial Press, 1999.

Butler, John Sibley. *Entrepreneurship and Self-Help among Black Americans: A Reconsideration of Race and Economics.* New York: State University of New York Press, 1991, 2005.

Caron, Simone M. *Who Chooses? American Reproductive History since 1830.* Gainesville: University Press of Florida, 2008.

Cayleff, Susan E. "Self-Help and the Patent Medicine Business." In *Women, Health, and Medicine in America: A Historical Handbook,* edited by Rima D. Apple, 311–336. New York: Garland, 1990.

Chunn, Dorothy E, Susan Boyd, and Hester Lessard. *Reaction and Resistance: Feminism, Law, and Social Change.* Vancouver, BC: UBC Press, 2007.

Clarke, Adele E. "Maverick Reproductive Scientists and the Production of Contraceptives, 1915–2000+." In *Bodies of Technology: Women's Involvement with Reproductive Medicine,* edited by Ann Rudinow Saetnan, Nelly Oudshoorn, and Marta Kirejczyk, 37–89. Columbus: Ohio University Press, 2000.

Cline, Rebecca J. Welch. "Small Group Communication in Health Care." In *Communication and Health: Systems and Application,* edited by Eileen Berline Ray and Lewis Donahew, 69–91. Hillsdale, NJ: Erlbaum, 1990.

Cobble, Dorothy Sue. *The Other Women's Movement: Workplace Justice and Social Rights in Modern America.* Princeton, NJ: Princeton University Press, 2004.

Cohen, Barbara. "The Zine Project: Writing with a Personal Perspective." *Language Arts* 82:2 (2006): 129–138.

Collins, Patricia Hill. *Black Feminist Thought: Knowledge, Consciousness, and the Politics of Empowerment.* Boston: Unwin Hyman, 1990.

Copelton, Denise A. "Menstrual Extraction, Abortion, and the Political Context of Feminist Self-Help." *Advances in Gender Research* 8 (2004): 129–164.

Coyle, Kelly, and Debra Grodin. "Self-Help Books and the Construction of Reading: Readers and Reading in Textual Representation." *Text and Performance Quarterly* 13 (1993): 61–78.

Craven, Christa. *Pushing for Midwives: Homebirth Mothers and the Reproductive Rights Movement.* Philadelphia: Temple University Press, 2010.

Davis, Kathy. *The Making of "Our Bodies, Ourselves": How Feminism Travels across Borders.* Durham, NC: Duke University Press, 2007.

Dicker, Rory Cooke, and Alison Piepmeier. *Catching a Wave: Reclaiming Feminism for the 21st Century.* Boston: Northeastern University Press, 2003.

Dreifus, Claudia. *Seizing Our Bodies: The Politics of Women's Health.* New York: Vintage Books, 1977.

Ebben, Maureen. "Off the Shelf Salvation: A Feminist Critique of Self-Help." *Women's Studies in Communication* 18:2 (1995): 111–122.

Echols, Alice. *Daring to Be Bad: Radical Feminism in America, 1967–1975.* Minneapolis: University of Minnesota Press, 1989.

Ehrenreich, Barbara, and Deirdre English. *For Her Own Good: 150 Years of the Experts' Advice to Women.* Garden City, NY: Anchor Press, 1978.

———. *Witches, Midwives, and Nurses: A History of Women Healers.* New York: Feminist Press at City University of New York, 1973.

Eichhorn, Kate. *The Archival Turn in Feminism: Outrage in Order.* Philadelphia: Temple University Press, 2013.

Enke, Anne. *Finding the Movement: Sexuality, Contested Space, and Women's Activism.* Durham, NC: Duke University Press, 2007.

Evans, Sara. *Personal Politics: The Roots of Women's Liberation in the Civil Rights Move-ment and the New Left.* New York: Knopf, 1979.

Fett, Sharla. *Working Cures: Healing, Health, and Power on Southern Slave Plantations.* Chapel Hill: University of North Carolina Press, 2002.

Fraser, Gertrude Jacinta. *African American Midwifery in the South: Dialogues of Birth, Race, and Memory.* Cambridge, MA: Harvard University Press, 1998.

Freeman, Jo. *The Politics of Women's Liberation: A Case Study of an Emerging Social Movement and Its Relation to the Policy Process.* New York: Addison-Wesley Longman, 1975.

———. "The Tyranny of Structurelessness." In *Dear Sisters: Dispatches from the Women's Liberation Movement,* edited by Rosalyn Baxandall and Linda Gordon, 73–75. New York: Basic Books, 2000.

Free to Choose: A Women's Guide to Reproductive Freedom. Portland, OR: Eberhardt Press, 2006.

Fried, Marlene Gerber. *From Abortion to Reproductive Freedom: Transforming a Move-ment.* Boston: South End Press, 1990.

Gachupin, Francine C., and Jennie Rose Joe. *Health and Social Issues of Native American Women.* Santa Barbara, CA: Praeger, 2012.

Gallagher, Dana, and Gary A. Richwald. "Feminism and Regulation Collide: The Food and Drug Administration's Approval of the Cervical Cap." *Women and Health* 15 (2009): 87–97.

Gerber, Susan. "The Evolving Gender Gap in General Obstetrics." *American Journal of Obstetrics and Gynecology* 195, no. 5 (2006): 1427–1430.

Gilmore, Stephanie. *Feminist Coalitions: Historical Perspectives on Second-Wave Feminism in the United States.* Urbana: University of Illinois Press, 2008.

———. *Groundswell: Grassroots Feminist Activism in Postwar America.* New York: Routledge, 2013.

Gordon, Linda. *The Moral Property of Women: A History of Birth Control Politics in America.* Urbana: University of Illinois Press, 2002.

Grodin, Debra. "The Interpreting Audience: The Therapeutics of Self-Help Book Reading." *Critical Studies in Mass Communication* 8 (1991): 404–420.

Gurr, Barbara. *Reproductive Justice: The Politics of Health Care for Native American Women.* New Brunswick, NJ: Rutgers University Press, 2015.

Guy-Sheftall, Beverly. *Words of Fire: An Anthology of African-American Feminist Thought.* New York: New York University Press, 1995.

Harding, Sandra. *The Science Question in Feminism.* Ithaca, NY: Cornell University Press, 1986.

Harrison, Cynthia Ellen. *On Account of Sex: The Politics of Women's Issues, 1945–1968.* Berkeley: University of California Press, 1988.

Hepburn, Cuca. *Alive and Well: A Lesbian Health Guide.* Freedom, CA: Crossing Press, 1988.

Hewitt, Nancy. *No Permanent Waves: Recasting Histories of U.S. Feminism.* New Brunswick, NJ: Rutgers University Press, 2010.

Heywood, Leslie. *The Women's Movement Today: An Encyclopedia of Third-Wave Feminism.* Westport, CT: Greenwood Press, 2006.

Heywood, Leslie, and Jennifer Drake. *Third Wave Agenda: Being Feminist, Doing Feminism.* Minneapolis: University of Minnesota Press, 1997.

Hogan, Kristen. *The Feminist Bookstore Movement: Lesbian Antiracism and Accountability.* Durham, NC: Duke University Press, 2016.

Holmes, Helen. *Issues in Reproductive Technology*. New York: New York University Press, 1992.

Holmes, Helen, Betty Hoskins, and Michael Gross. *Birth Control and Controlling Birth: Women-Centered Perspectives*. Clifton, NJ: Humana Press, 1980.

Hornstein, Francie. "Children by Donor Insemination: A New Choice for Lesbians." In *Test Tube Women: What Future for Motherhood?*, edited by Rita Arditti, Renate Duelli Klein, and Shelley Minden, 356–370. Boston: Pandora Press, 1984.

Houck, Judith. *Hot and Bothered: Women, Medicine, and Menopause in Modern America*. Cambridge: Harvard University Press, 2008.

Houck, Judith A. "The Best Prescription for Women's Health: Feminist Approaches to Well-Woman Care." In *Prescribed: Writing, Filling, Using, and Abusing the Prescription in Modern America*, edited by Jeremy Greene and Elizabeth Siegel Watkins, 134–156. Baltimore: Johns Hopkins University Press, 2012.

Huckle, Patricia. *Tish Sommers, Activist, and the Founding of the Older Women's League*. Knoxville: University of Tennessee Press, 1991.

Huff, Cynthia. *Women's Life Writing and Imagined Communities*. New York: Routledge, 2005.

Iannello, Kathleen P. *Decisions without Hierarchy: Feminist Interventions in Organization Theory and Practice*. New York: Routledge, 1992.

Jaimes, M. Annette. *The State of Native America: Genocide, Colonization, and Resistance*. Boston: South End Press, 1992.

Joffe, Carole E. *Dispatches from the Abortion Wars: The Costs of Fanaticism to Doctors, Patients, and the Rest of Us*. Boston: Beacon Press, 2009.

———. *Doctors of Conscience: The Struggle to Provide Abortion before and after Roe v. Wade*. Boston: Beacon Press, 1995.

Johnson, Merri Lisa. *Third Wave Feminism and Television: Jane Puts It in a Box*. New York: Palgrave Macmillan, 2007.

Kaplan, Laura. *The Story of Jane: The Legendary Underground Feminist Abortion Service*. Chicago: University of Chicago Press, 1995.

Katz, Alfred H. *Self-Help in America: A Social Movement Perspective*. New York: Twayne, 1993.

Klein, Ethel. *Gender Politics: From Consciousness to Mass Politics*. Cambridge, MA: Harvard University Press, 1984.

Klein, Renate Duelli. "Doing It Ourselves: Self Insemination." In *Test Tube Women: What Future for Motherhood?*, edited by Rita Arditti, Renate Duelli Klein, and Shelley Minden, 382–390. Boston: Pandora Press, 1984.

Kline, Kimberly. "The Discursive Characteristics of a Prosocial Self-Help: Re-visioning the Potential of Self-Help for Empowerment." *Southern Communication Journal* 74 (2009): 191–208.

Kline, Wendy. *Bodies of Knowledge: Sexuality, Reproduction, and Women's Health in the Second Wave*. Chicago: University of Chicago Press, 2010.

———. "'Please Include This in Your Book': Readers Respond to *Our Bodies, Ourselves*." *Bulletin of the History of Medicine* 79:1 (2005): 81–110.

Kluchin, Rebecca M. "Pregnant? Need Help? Call Jane: Service as Radical Action in the Abortion Underground in Chicago." In *Breaking the Wave: Women, Their Organizations, and Feminism, 1945–1985*, edited by Kathleen A. Laughlin and Jaqueline L. Castledine, 136–154. New York: Routledge, 2011.

Kroløkke, Charlotte, and Ann Scott Sørensen. *Gender Communication Theories and Analyses: From Silence to Performance*. Thousand Oaks, CA: Sage, 2006.

Laughlin, Kathleen A., et al. "Is It Time to Jump Ship? Historians Rethink the Waves Metaphor." *Feminist Formations* 22:1 (2010): 76–135.

Lawrence, Jane. "The Indian Health Service and the Sterilization of Native American Women." *American Indian Quarterly* 24:3 (2000): 400–419.

Layne, Linda. "The Home Pregnancy Test: A Feminist Technology?" *Women's Studies Quarterly* 37:1 (2009): 61–79.

Layne, Linda, Sharra Louise Vostral, and Kate Boyer. *Feminist Technology*. Urbana: University of Illinois Press, 2010.

Leavitt, Judith Walzer. *Brought to Bed: Childbearing in America, 1750–1950*. New York: Oxford University Press, 1986.

———. *Make Room for Daddy: The Journey from Waiting Room to Birthing Room*. Chapel Hill: University of North Carolina Press, 2009.

———. "'A Private Little Revolution': The Home Pregnancy Test in American Culture." *Bulletin of the History of Medicine* 80:2 (2006): 317–345.

Lichterman, Paul. "Self-Help Reading as a Thin Culture." *Media, Culture, and Society* 14 (1992): 421–447.

Luce, Jacquelyne. *Beyond Expectation: Lesbian/Bi/Queer Women and Assisted Conception*. Toronto: University of Toronto Press, 2010.

Luker, Kristin. *Abortion and the Politics of Motherhood*. Berkeley: University of California Press, 1984.

Mamo, Laura. *Queering Reproduction: Achieving Pregnancy in the Age of Technoscience*. Durham, NC: Duke University Press, 2007.

Marieskind, Helen. "Helping Oneself to Health." *Social Policy* 7 (1976): 63–66.

Marieskind, Helen, and Barbara Ehrenreich. "Toward a Socialist Medicine: The Women's Health Movement." *Social Policy* 6 (1975): 34–42.

Matthews, Holly F. "Killing the Medical Self-Help Tradition among African Americans: The Case of Lay Midwifery in North Carolina, 1912–1983." In *African Americans in the South: Issues of Race, Class, and Gender*, edited by Hans Baer and Yvonne Jones, 60–78. Athens: University of Georgia Press, 1992.

Mayeri, Serena. *Reasoning from Race: Feminism, Law, and the Civil Rights Movement*. Cambridge, MA: Harvard University Press, 2011.

Mays, Vickie. "Black Women, Work, Stress, and Perceived Discrimination: The Focused Support Group Model as an Intervention for Stress Reduction." *Cultural Diversity and Mental Health* 1 (1995): 53–65.

Michaels, Paula. *Lamaze: An International History*. Oxford: Oxford University Press, 2014.

Mizrahi, Terry. "Women's Ways of Organizing: Strengths and Struggles of Women Activists over Time." *Affilia: Journal of Women and Social Work* 22:1 (2007): 39–55.

Morgen, Sandra. *Into Our Own Hands: The Women's Health Movement in the United States, 1969–1990*. New Brunswick, NJ: Rutgers University Press, 2002.

Murphy, Michelle. "Immodest Witnessing: The Epistemology of Vaginal Self-Examination in the U.S. Feminist Self-Help Movement." *Feminist Studies* 30 (2004): 115–147.

———. *Seizing the Means of Reproduction: Entanglements of Feminism, Health, and Technoscience*. Durham, NC: Duke University Press, 2012.

Nelson, Jennifer. "'All This That Has Happened to Me Shouldn't Happen to Nobody Else': Loretta Ross and the Women of Color Reproductive Freedom Movement of the 1980s." *Journal of Women's History* 22:3 (2010): 136–160.

———. *More Than Medicine: A History of the Feminist Women's Health Movement*. New York: New York University Press, 2015.

——. *Women of Color and the Reproductive Rights Movement.* New York: New York University Press, 2003.

Orleck, Annalise. *Storming Caesar's Palace: How Black Mothers Fought Their Own War on Poverty.* Boston: Beacon Press, 2005.

Piepmeier, Alison. *Girl Zines: Making Media, Doing Feminism.* New York: New York University Press, 2009.

Ralstin-Lewis, D. Marie. "The Continuing Struggle against Genocide: Indigenous Women's Reproductive Rights." *Wicazo Sa Review* 20:1 (2005): 71–95.

Rapping, Elayne. *The Culture of Recovery: Making Sense of the Self-Help Movement in Women's Lives.* Boston: Beacon Press, 1996.

——. "There's Self-Help and Then There's Self-Help: Women and the Recovery Movement." *Social Policy* 27:3 (1997): 56–61.

Reagan, Leslie. "Crossing the Border for Abortions: California Activists, Mexican Clinics, and the Creation of a Feminist Health Agency in the 1960s." *Feminist Studies* 26:2 (2000): 323–348.

——. *When Abortion Was a Crime: Women, Medicine, and the Law in the United States, 1867–1973.* Berkeley: University of California Press, 1998.

Reger, Jo. *Everywhere and Nowhere: Contemporary Feminism in the United States.* New York: Oxford University Press, 2012.

Rife, James P., and Alan J. Dellapenna. *Caring and Curing: A History of the Indian Health Service.* Terra Alta, WV: PHS Commissioner Officers Foundation for the Advancement of Public Health, 2009.

Ristock, Janice, "Feminist Collectives: The Struggles and Contradictions in Our Quest for a 'Uniquely Feminist Structure.'" In *Women and Social Change: Feminist Activism in Canada*, edited by Jeri Wine and Janice Ristock, 41–55. Halifax: James Lorimer and Company, 1991.

Roberts, Dorothy. *Killing the Black Body: Race, Reproduction, and the Meaning of Liberty.* New York: Pantheon Books, 1997.

Roberts, Lynn, Loretta Ross, and M. Bahati Kuumba. "The Reproductive Health and Sexual Rights of Women of Color: Still Building a Movement." *NWSA Journal* 17:1 (2005): 93–98.

Roepke, Clare L., and Eric A. Schaff. "Long Tail Strings: Impact of the Dalkon Shield 40 Years Later." *Open Journal of Obstetrics and Gynecology* 4 (2014): 996–1005.

Rose, Melody. *Safe, Legal, and Unavailable? Abortion Politics in the United States.* Washington, DC: CQ Press, 2007.

Rosen, Ruth. *The World Split Open: How the Modern Women's Movement Changed America.* New York: Penguin Books, 2000.

Ross, Jeffrey Ian. *American Indians at Risk.* Santa Barbara, CA: ABC-CLIO, 2014.

Ross, Loretta, and Rickie Solinger. *Reproductive Justice: An Introduction.* Oakland: University of California Press, 2017.

Ross, Loretta, et al. *Radical Reproductive Justice: Foundation, Theory, Practice, Critique.* New York: Feminist Press at the City University of New York, 2017.

Roth, Benita. *Separate Roads to Feminism: Black, Chicana, and White Feminist Movements in America's Second Wave.* New York: Cambridge University Press, 2004.

Ruzek, Sheryl Burk. *The Women's Health Movement: Feminist Alternatives to Medical Control.* New York: Praeger, 1978.

Ryan, Barbara. *Feminism and the Women's Movement: Dynamics of Change in Social Movement Ideology, and Activism.* New York: Routledge, 1992.

Sandelowski, Margaret. "'The Most Dangerous Instrument': Propriety, Power, and the Vaginal Speculum." *Journal of Obstetric, Gynecological and Neonatal Nursing* 29:1 (2000): 73–82.

Sarachild, Kathie. "Consciousness Raising: A Radical Weapon." In *Feminist Revolution*. Edited by Redstockings. New York: Random House, 1975.

Schoen, Johanna. *Abortion after Roe: Abortion after Legalization*. Chapel Hill: University of North Carolina Press, 2015.

———. *Choice and Coercion: Birth Control, Sterilization, and Abortion in Public Health and Welfare*. Chapel Hill: University of North Carolina Press, 2005.

———. "Reconceiving Abortion: Medical Practice, Women's Access, and Feminist Politics before and after *Roe v. Wade*." *Feminist Studies* 26:2 (2000): 349–376.

Schrager, Cynthia D. "Questioning the Promise of Self-Help: A Reading of 'Women Who Love Too Much.'" *Feminist Studies* 19 (1993): 176–192.

Seaman, Barbara, and Laura Eldridge. *Voices of the Women's Health Movement*. Vol. 1. New York: Seven Stories Press, 2012.

Shodhini. *Touch Me, Touch Me Not: Women, Plants, and Healing*. New Delhi: Kali for Women, 1997.

Siegel, Deborah. *Sisterhood, Interrupted: From Radical Women to Grrls Gone Wild*. New York: Palgrave Macmillan, 2007.

Silliman, Jael, et al. *Undivided Rights: Women of Color Organize for Reproductive Justice*. Cambridge, MA: South End Press, 2004.

Simonds, Wendy. *Abortion at Work: Ideology and Practice in a Feminist Clinic*. New Brunswick, NJ: Rutgers University Press, 1996.

———. *Women and Self-Help Culture: Reading between the Lines*. New Brunswick, NJ: Rutgers University Press, 1992.

Smith, Andrea. *Conquest: Sexual Violence and American Indian Genocide*. Cambridge, MA: South End Press, 2005.

Smith, Barbara. *Home Girls: A Black Feminist Anthology*. New Brunswick, NJ: Kitchen Table—Women of Color Press, 1983.

Smith, Susan L. *Sick and Tired of Being Sick and Tired: Women's Health Activism in America, 1890–1950*. Philadelphia: University of Pennsylvania Press, 1995.

Solinger, Rickie. *Abortion Wars: A Half Century of Struggle, 1950–2000*. Los Angeles: University of California Press, 1998.

———. *Wake Up Little Susie: Single Pregnancy and Race before Roe v. Wade*. New York: Routledge, 2000.

Spain, Daphne. *Constructive Feminism: Women's Spaces and Women's Rights in the American City*. Ithaca, NY: Cornell University Press, 2016.

Staggenborg, Suzanne. *The Pro-choice Movement: Organization and Activism in the Abortion Conflict*. New York: Oxford University Press, 1991.

Stoderling, Stina, and Alison Bernstein. "Dazon Dixon Diallo: Feminism and the Fight to Combat HIV/AIDS." In *Junctures in Women's Leadership: Social Movements*, edited by Mary Trigg and Alison Bernstein 161–176. New Brunswick, NJ: Rutgers University Press, 2016.

Strobel, Margaret. "Organizational Learning in the Chicago Women's Liberation Union." In *Feminist Organizations: Harvest of the New Women's Movement*, edited by Myra Ferree and Patricia Martin, 145–164. Philadelphia: Temple University Press, 1995.

Taylor, Verta. *Rock-a-by Baby: Feminism, Self-Help and Postpartum Depression*. New York: Routledge, 1996.

Thompson, Becky. "Multiracial Feminism: Recasting the Chronology of Second Wave Feminism." *Feminist Studies* 28:2 (2002): 336–360.

Thorn, Mary. *Inside Ms.: 25 Years of the Magazine and the Feminist Movement*. New York: Holt, 1997.

Tone, Andrea. *Devices and Desires: A History of Contraceptives in America*. New York: Hill and Wang, 2001.

Tunc, Tanfer Emin. "Innovators and Instigators: Feminist Contributions to American Abortion Technology, 1963–1973." *Journal of Family Planning and Reproductive Healthcare* 33:3 (August 2007): 149–154.

Ulrich, Laurel Thatcher. *A Midwife's Tale: The Life of Martha Ballard, Based on Her Diary, 1785–1812*. New York: Vintage Books, 1990.

Valk, Anne M. *Radical Sisters: Second-Wave Feminism and Black Liberation in Washington, D.C.* Urbana: University of Illinois Press, 2008.

Van Zoonen, Liesbet. "Gendering the Internet: Claims, Controversies, and Cultures." *European Journal of Communication* 17:1 (2002): 5–23.

Vostral, Sharra Louise. *Under Wraps: A History of Menstrual Hygiene Technology*. Lanham, MD: Lexington Books, 2008.

Wajcman, Judy. *Feminism Confronts Technology*. University Park: Pennsylvania State University Press, 1991.

———. "TechnoCapitalism Meets Technofeminism: Women and Technology in a Wireless World." *Labour and Industry* 16:3 (2006): 7–20.

Wanggren, Kjell, et al. "Teaching Medical Students Gynaecological Examination Using Professional Patients: Evaluation of Students' Skills and Feelings." *Medical Teacher* 27:2 (2005): 130–135.

Warsh, Cheryl Krasnick. *Prescribed Norms: Women and Health in Canada and the United States since 1800*. North York, ON: University of Toronto Press, 2010.

Wells, Susan. *Our Bodies, Ourselves, and the Work of Writing*. Stanford, CA: Stanford University Press, 2010.

Wertz, Richard W., and Dorothy C. Wertz. *Lying-In: A History of Childbirth in America*. New Haven, CT: Yale University Press, 1989.

White, Evelyn. *Black Women's Health Book: Speaking for Ourselves*. Seattle: Seal Press, 1994.

White, Jocelyn, and Marissa C. Martinez. *The Lesbian Health Book: Caring for Ourselves*. Seattle: Seal Press, 1997.

Winthorn, Ann. "Helping Ourselves: The Limits and Potential of Self-Help." *Social Policy* 11:3 (1980): 20–27.

Wolf, Jacqueline H. *Deliver Me from Pain: Anesthesia and Birth in America*. Baltimore: Johns Hopkins University Press, 2011.

Wolf, Susan. *Feminism and Bioethics: Beyond Reproduction*. New York: Oxford University Press, 1996.

Index